VITAMINS AGAINST CANCER

VITAMINS AGAINST CANCER

Fact and Fiction

Dr. Kedar N. Prasad

Healing Arts Press
Rochester, Vermont

Healing Arts Press
One Park Street
Rochester, Vermont 05767

LIBRARY OF CONGRESS CATALOGING-IN-PUBLICATION DATA

Prasad, Kedar N.
Vitamins against cancer / by Kedar N. Prasad.
p.   cm.
Reprint. Originally published: Denver, Colo. : Nutrition Pub.
House, c1984.
Bibliography: p.
Includes index.
ISBN 0-89281-294-X
1. Cancer—Diet therapy.   2. Vitamin therapy. 3. Cancer—
Nutritional aspects.   I. Title.
[RC271.D52P73   1989]
616.99'40654—dc19   88-33071
CIP

Printed and bound in the United States

10 9 8 7 6 5 4 3 2 1

Healing Arts Press is a division of Inner Traditions International, Ltd.

Distributed to the book trade in the United States by Harper and Row
Publishers, Inc.

Distributed to the book trade in Canada by Book Center, Inc.,
Montreal, Quebec

Distributed to the health food trade in Canada by Alive Books,
Toronto and Vancouver

Contents

Contents

ABOUT THE AUTHOR

Dr. Kedar N. Prasad is an internationally recognized authority on vitamins, nutrition and cancer. He has published over 150 original research articles on the biology of cancer cells in internationally known scientific journals and has written and edited several books on cancer. He is the editor of the book *Vitamins, Nutrition and Cancer* and coeditor of the book *Modulation and Mediation of Cancer by Vitamins* (both available through Karger Press, Basel, Switzerland). Dr. Prasad has delivered numerous lectures on vitamins, nutrition and cancer all over the world. He has also organized international meetings in order to increase the exchange of information in this area between scientists of different countries.

Dr. Prasad is a member of several major national and international scientific societies. At present he is president of the International Association for Vitamin and Nutritional Oncology. He is currently a professor in the Department of Radiology and Director of the Center for Vitamins and Cancer Research at the School of Medicine, University of Colorado Health Sciences Center, Denver, Colorado 80262, USA.

Preface

An increasing number of people interested in improving and maintaining their health are using supplementary nutrition to achieve their goals. Recent studies estimate that about 40 percent of the people in the United States use some form of supplementary nutrition every day. Most of them are unaware of recent developments concerning nutrition and cancer, and many may be taking nutrients without using up-to-date scientific guidelines. It is well known that excessive consumption of certain nutrients can cause irreversible damage to the body.

This book has two major purposes: (1) To make the public aware of the results of recent research on vitamins, nutrition and cancer; and (2) to provide interim guidelines which can be used to develop individual dietary and supplementary nutritional programs for cancer prevention and treatment. Such programs must be developed in close consultation with physicians who are knowledgeable about nutrition and cancer. The cancer prevention program may be equally effective for maintaining good health. Also included are a list of major scientific publications on vitamins, nutrition and cancer, and an international list of over 100 major institutions where vitamins and nutrition are being used in the prevention and treatment of cancer.

Foreword

The lay public has become increasingly interested in monitoring personal health and has been besieged with recommendations from many different organizations and individuals. A particularly controversial area has been that of vitamins and cancer. Dr. Prasad has prepared a useful and well organized antidote to the mass of irresponsible information about vitamins. He opens with a short, clever review of what is "fact and fiction" about vitamins and cancer; this perspective alone is worth the purchase of the book.

The author then presents in logical fashion the potential role of vitamins in the prevention and treatment of human cancer. His review of laboratory and epidemiological evidence for vitamins as natural inhibitors of cancer is well presented and understandable to the average individual. His interim guidelines for vitamin usage, diet changes and lifestyle considerations for the prevention of human cancer are considered and reasonable. The distinction between the doses of vitamins and nutrients that may be necessary for adequate nutrition versus cancer prevention is an important issue and one which he presents in a balanced fashion.

Major new areas of research on the potential role of vitamins in the treatment of cancer or in alleviating the effects of treatment for cancer are discussed. The author's presentation of this rapidly developing field is well balanced, and research results are viewed with cautious optimism.

Finally, the list of more than one hundred internationally recognized clinical and laboratory investigators in the area of vitamins, nutrition and cancer is extremely valuable and one which we hope will be used by the public.

As a physician who frequently sees bad results from the misuse of vitamins for nutrition or prevention or treatment of human cancer, I applaud Dr. Prasad for providing the public with a responsible presentation.

Frank L. Meyskens, Jr., M.D.
Director, University of California Cancer Center
Route 88, 101 City Drive
Orange, CA 92668

CHAPTER

1.

What is Fact and What is Fiction?

A BRIEF DISCUSSION

During the last few years, many popular magazines and books have described new advances in vitamin and nutrition research. Unfortunately, many of these reports have made unsubstantiated claims regarding the usefulness of nutrition for maintaining good health and preventing cancer. As a result, a number of misconceptions have arisen concerning the value of nutrition. Some beliefs commonly held by the general public are discussed below.

1. **FICTION:** The more vitamins and other supplementary nutrients you take, the better you will feel.

    FACT: *This belief can be dangerous. Consumption of excessive amounts of certain nutrients may cause severe damage. For instance, taking large amounts of vitamin A (50,000 I.U.[1] or more per day over a long period of time) may cause liver toxicity, and excessive selenium (500 micrograms or more per day over a long period of time) may cause cataracts (an eye disease in which the lens becomes opaque).*

2. **FICTION:** All the different forms of vitamins A, C or E are similar and produce similar effects.

---

[1] I.U. = International Unit.

1

FACT: *The above statement is untrue. For example, some of the actions of beta-carotene and retinol (both forms of vitamin A) are different. Similarly, vitamin E (alpha-tocopherol) can act as an antioxidant, whereas vitamin E acetate (alpha-tocopherol acetate) and vitamin E succinate (alpha-tocopherol succinate) do not. Although there is only one form of vitamin C, it is commonly prepared in combination with several minerals. Vitamin C preparations containing iron, manganese and copper may be harmful, because vitamin C in the presence of these metals and oxygen produces toxic substances. Vitamin C preparations containing sodium, magnesium and calcium have no such effects.*

3. **FICTION:** Frozen fruit juices and powdered cold drinks after being mixed with water maintain high levels of vitamin C when stored in a refrigerator.

    FACT: *This statement is also untrue. Frozen fruit juices and powdered cold drinks may provide beneficial amounts of vitamin C when drunk immediately after preparation. However, when it is stored in a cold place, vitamin C in solution rapidly deteriorates, and after 24 hours more than 50 percent of its activity is lost.*

4. **FICTION:** Some people believe that to maintain good health or prevent cancer, they can take all their vitamins once in the morning with breakfast; others believe that taking vitamins once in a while, especially during cold weather, is enough.

    FACT: *These beliefs are incorrect. The frequency with which one should take vitamins depends upon their rate of degradation in the body. Taking vitamins A and E orally twice a day (morning and evening) is adequate; this is not the case with vitamin C. Vitamin C is degraded rapidly in the body (usually within 2–4 hours); thus it is recommended that vitamin C be consumed at least 4 times a day. In addition, for cancer prevention, the consumption of vitamins at the appropriate time, depending on one's diet, is very important. Taking* *supplementary vitamins once in a while has no real health value.*

5. **FICTION**: Avoiding excessive meat consumption is not relevant to preventing cancer.

    FACT: *Wrong. Excessive consumption of meat in the Western countries has been linked with colon cancer. This is further supported by the fact that the incidence of colon cancer among Seventh Day Adventists, who are vegetarians, is also low.*

6. **FICTION**: Supplementary nutrition is not necessary for cancer prevention.

    FACT: *Results of recent studies on human beings are not sufficient to fully support or reject the above view. However, there are a number of animal studies which suggest that supplementary nutrition is essential in preventing cancer.*

7. **FICTION**: A balanced diet is sufficient for optimal protection against cancer.

    FACT: *The concept of a "balanced diet" is very general. A balanced diet alone may not be adequate for optimal protection against cancer, although it is certainly better than a junk food diet. It is also important to take vitamins A, C and E at appropriate times, such as when one consumes food which contains cancer-causing substances. It may not be possible or practical to receive the required levels of these vitamins at the appropriate times only through a balanced diet. For these reasons, supplementary nutrition, in addition to a balanced diet, is essential for maximal protection against cancer.*

8. **FICTION**: Our environment and our food and water are already polluted, and none of us can do anything about it. Therefore, we have to accept the increasing risk of cancer as a reality.

    FACT: *Even though we cannot do very much immediately to remove cancer-causing substances from our environment and diet, we can certainly reduce their cancer-causing actions through proper food, supplementary nutrition and lifestyle.*

9. **FICTION**: An excess of zinc is necessary for maximal

health and cancer prevention.

FACT: *This may not be true. Actually, excessive zinc may block the action of selenium, an important anticancer agent.*

10. **FICTION:** Cancer is a disease of old people, so you don't have to worry about a child's nutrition as a preventive measure.

    FACT: *This may be true for some cancers, such as colon and rectal cancer. However, most cancers can occur at any age. Thus, for preventing cancer, proper nutrition is equally important for children.*

11. **FICTION:** There is no scientific proof that supplementary vitamins are any good.

    FACT: *The effectiveness of supplementary vitamins in preventing cancer and maintaining sound health has not been fully established in human beings. It will take 40 to 50 years before conclusive results become available. However, laboratory studies suggest vitamins can strengthen the body's immune defense system, reduce levels of cancer-causing substances, protect vital organs against the injurious effects of free radicals (harmful chemicals), block the action of cancer-causing substances, and suppress the growth of some kinds of cancer. Some of these benefits of vitamins have also been scientifically demonstrated in human beings.*

12. **FICTION:** Most supplementary vitamins pass out of the body in the urine and feces, so why take them?

    FACT: *At this time we do not know what dose of vitamins is needed for maximum cancer prevention and maintaining sound health. The dietary vitamin E is present as mixed tocopherols which act as an antioxidant, but they are unstable. The commercially made alpha-tocopheryl acetate is stable, but it does not act as an antioxidant until converted to alpha-tocopherol in the body. The turnover rate of vitamin C in the body is fairly rapid, so it is not practical to take vitamin C in foods frequently enough to maintain sustained high levels in the body. Some excess amounts of vitamin C and vitamin*

E (alpha-tocopherol) are needed in the stomach to reduce levels of nitrosamines, potent cancer-causing agents, if nitrite-containing foods such as bacon, sausage, hot dogs and cured meats are eaten. The presence of these vitamins is necessary at the time such foods are consumed. Since we do not know the quantities of vitamins needed by the cells, it is important to give them the opportunity to pick up the amounts they need. Thus, even though significant amounts of supplementary vitamins are excreted in the feces and urine, they may have already performed an important role in the body by then. For this reason, excess amounts of vitamins in the feces and urine should not be considered wasteful.

13. **FICTION:** Supplementary vitamin C causes kidney stones.

    FACT: *This effect has not been observed in average normal adults. It is well established that if the urine becomes acidic, some of the waste products in the kidney may solidify and form "stones." However, this biological phenomenon usually occurs if there is an imbalance in body chemistry such that acidic solutions cannot be neutralized. The body normally has a tremendous capacity to neutralize any acidic solution which it takes in. In certain specific disease conditions in which one's body has lost this capacity, one should not take vitamin C in acid form.*

14. **FICTION:** Supplementary vitamins are addictive.

    FACT: *Although high doses of vitamin C (up to 20 grams per day) have been used in treating heroin addiction, they have not caused permanent addictive changes in the body. However, persons who are taking high doses of supplementary vitamins should not stop abruptly. Because body systems may have adjusted to high doses of vitamins, sudden withdrawal may cause symptoms of vitamin deficiency.*

15. **FICTION:** Vitamins and nutrients alone are sufficient to treat all cancers.

    FACT: *Because of the complexities of cancer, neither vitamins* *nor any other agents can cure advanced tumors by themselves, but vitamins may be very useful in combination with other kinds of therapy. Vitamins may also help delay or prevent the recurrence of cancer. Using vitamins to treat cancer must be done according to scientific rationale; to use them otherwise may be ineffective.*

At this time, vitamins A, C and E are used as experimental drugs, either alone or in combination with other conventional treatment methods. The results of these studies are not completely known at this time. Therefore, until better methods of cancer treatment are established, the utilization of all current treatment methods must be continued.

CHAPTER

2.

Preventing Cancer

WHAT CAUSES CANCER?

What are cancer cells? Cancer cells divide like some normal cells, but unlike normal cells they continue to divide without any restriction and invade distant organs in the body. When normal cells are grown outside the body in laboratory petri dishes, a procedure known as tissue culture,* they have a limited lifespan, and all of them eventually die even when they have nutrients and space. In this sense normal cells can be considered "mortal," whereas cancer cells are "immortal." Cancer cells will continue to grow in petri dishes indefinitely, provided sufficient nutrients and space are available.

Cancer can arise in any organ containing dividing cells (e.g., bone marrow, skin, intestine and testes) or having cells which normally do not divide but which will divide if properly stimulated (e.g., liver cells, glia cells in the brain).

Certain tumors occur primarily among children. These include neuroblastoma (in the abdominal cavity), Wilms' tumor (in the kidney), medulloblastoma (in the brain), retinoblastoma (in the eye), and some types of leukemia (blood cancer). On the other hand, colon and rectal cancers are found primarily in persons over 50 years of age. Most other cancers

---

*Tissue culture is a method by which cells are grown in laboratory dishes containing adequate nutrients. This method is commonly used in cancer research because it is simple, sensitive, cost-effective and efficient.

can occur at any age. Cancers not only affect human beings and other mammals but also occur in lower organisms such as reptiles, frogs, fish, snails and clams.

How do normal cells become cancerous? It is now believed that all normal cells have cancer genes* (called oncogenes), but that they do not exert their influence until activated by cancer-causing agents. The products of these activated genes may convert one or more normal cells to cancer cells. Agents which activate cancer genes are called *tumor initiators*. High doses of *tumor initiators* by themselves can produce cancer; low doses of tumor initiators cannot cause cancer unless they are helped by other agents called *tumor promoters*. Even high doses of tumor promoters generally do not produce cancer, but with prolonged exposure they may also be carcinogenic.

Human beings are seldom exposed to high doses of tumor initiators or promoters, but they are frequently exposed to low doses of these cancer-causing substances. Subsequent cancer-initiated events may remain dormant for 10–30 years or more, until further genetic changes occur, and can appear as cancer cells if helped by other initiators or tumor promoters. Laboratory experiments have shown that the combined influence of two initiators is more effective than the individual agents in producing cancer. Some commonly known tumor initiators and tumor promoters are listed in Table 1. Most of these are found in the environment and diet (see pages 17–20 for a detailed description).

---

*DNA (deoxyribonucleic acid) molecules, also referred to as genes, are present in all cells. Segments of genes responsible for increasing the risk of cancer are called oncogenes (cancer-causing genes).

TABLE 1
Commonly Known Tumor Initiators
and Promoters

Tumor Initiators	Tumor Promoters
Nitrosamine	Saccharine
7,12-Dimethylbenz(a) anthracene (DMBA)	Excess fat
Benzopyrene	Croton oil
Ionizing radiation (X rays and gamma rays)	Citrus oil
Ultraviolet radiation	12-O-tetradecanoyl-phorbol-13-acetate
Asbestos	High temperatures (43°–45 °C, or 109.4°–111 °F)
Pesticides (malathion, parathion, kepone, DDT)	Certain hormones such as estrogen and epidermal growth factors
Tobacco smoke	Extract of unburned tobacco
Diethylstilbestrol (DES)	Tobacco smoke condensate
Aflatoxin	Surface active agents (sodium lauryl sulfate)
Polychlorinated biphenyl (PCB)	Iodoacetic acid

(Table 1, continued)

Polyvinyl chloride (PVC)	Phenobarbital
Certain heavy metals such as lead, mercury and arsenic compounds	Sex steroids
Tannic acid	Teleocidin, isolated from herbs, *Streptomyces mediocidicus*

What is the rate of cancer in the United States? It has been estimated that one of every four Americans will develop some form of cancer. Since the current population of the United States is about 245 million, the total number of people now alive in this country who will develop cancer is about 61 million. Projected figures for 1988 show that approximately 985,000 new cases of cancer were diagnosed, and approximately 494,000 people died of cancer. After cardiovascular disease, cancer is the second most common cause of death in the United States.

How much do diet and other environmental factors contribute to the incidence of cancer? It has been estimated that 70–80 percent of all human cancers are induced by environmental factors; 30–40 percent of these in men, and 50–60 percent in women, are thought to result from diet alone. Most of these cancers can be prevented by choosing a suitable diet, by taking appropriate amounts of nutritional supplements, by altering one's lifestyle, and by reducing the consumption of dietary and environmental cancer-causing substances as much as possible.

The relationship of diet and lifestyle to cancer has been observed in many parts of the world. Some examples are given below.

Table 2 shows the incidence of death associated with certain types of cancer.

TABLE 2

The Percentage of Deaths From Cancer of Different Parts of the Body Differs in Men and Women

Cancer Site	Male	Female
	(% of total cancer deaths)	
Lung	34	16
Colon and rectum	12	15
Prostate	10	—
Breast	0	19
Female reproductive organs (ovary, uterus and cervix)	—	11

Based on current estimates

Japan

A high incidence of stomach cancer has been associated with the consumption of spices and pickled food. The rate of stomach cancer is markedly reduced among those Japanese immigrants who adopt Western food habits; however, the incidence of stomach cancer remains high among Japanese immigrants to the United States who continue to follow Japanese dietary habits.

Chile

The high incidence of stomach cancer in Chile appears to be associated with consumption of food and drinking water that contain relatively high levels of nitrate, a chemical that combines with other chemicals (amines) in the stomach to form nitrosamine, a highly potent cancer-causing substance.

Iceland
The incidence of stomach cancer among Icelanders who consume large quantities of smoked fish and meat is much higher than among those who eat such food in smaller amounts.

India
The high incidence of oral cancer in India is associated with chewing betel nuts containing several cancer-causing agents. The habit of holding dry tobacco leaves between the lip and gum is associated with a high incidence of lip cancer. The latter is not unique to India, but is common to all regions where people chew tobacco in the manner described above.

Colon cancer is virtually absent among the Punjabi people in northwest India, who eat a diet rich in cellulose, vegetables, fiber and yogurt.

United States
The incidence of stomach cancer has decreased recently because of changing dietary habits. The rate of colon and rectal cancer among Seventh Day Adventists who eat a vegetarian diet is much less than among those who eat meat. In addition, Mormons, who do not smoke or drink alcohol or large quantities of coffee, have a lower incidence of colon and rectal cancer.

China
In one province of China, people have a very high incidence of esophageal cancer. The high incidence of this cancer appears to be related to the fact that the selenium (an anticancer nutrient) content of the soil is very low. The people of

this region eat mostly pickled food and only small quantities of fruits and vegetables.

What happens when meat is cooked over charcoal? During warm weather, broiling meat over charcoal is a popular practice; however, recent studies suggest that this practice may increase the risk of cancer. On the other hand, if it is done in moderation and with scientific rationale, the possibility of such risk may be markedly reduced. To understand this, let us examine what happens when meat is cooked over charcoal.

As the meat cooks, fats drip down onto the hot charcoal, generating smoke which contains polycyclic aromatic hydrocarbons, such as benzopyrene, a powerful cancer-causing agent. The cooking meat is immediately exposed to and absorbs this smoke. Thus, charcoal-broiled meat contains carcinogenic substances from the smoke and noncharcoal-broiled meat does not. The amount of polycyclic aromatic hydrocarbons increases if the fat content of the meat is high and if it is cooked under conditions that expose it to high levels of fat-generated smoke. It is estimated that the average charcoal-broiled steak contains about 8 micrograms of polycyclic aromatic hydrocarbons per kilogram of steak.

In order to reduce the levels of cancer-causing substances in charcoal-broiled meat, the fat should be removed as much as possible before cooking. In addition, the meat may be placed a little farther away from the charcoal during cooking so that at least part of the fat-generated smoke will dissipate into the air before it can reach the meat. Covering the grill with aluminum foil before placing meat on it will also prevent smoke contamination. It is important for the cook and others to avoid inhaling the smoke. The quality of the prepared meat will in no way be compromised by following these recommendations.

What goes on in your body when you smoke? Many studies have implicated tobacco smoking as a major cause of lung cancer, and 90 percent of all lung cancer cases are estimated to be caused by cigarette smoking. It has been reported that lung cancer accounts for 25 percent of all cancer deaths in the United States. In addition, smoking tobacco can cause chronic emphysema, a serious non-cancer disease, with severe effects on the functioning of the lungs. Cigarette smoke contains a high level of nitrosamine, a potent cancer-causing agent, and nitrosating gases, which help form additional nitrosamines in the lungs. Nitrosamines are easily dissolved in water and can thus be absorbed through the mouth as well as the lung and deposited in other organs. Smoking also increases the risk of developing cancer of the larynx, mouth and esophagus, and acts as a contributing factor for cancer of the urinary bladder, cervix, kidney and pancreas.

Some studies have reported that smoking decreases the tissue levels of vitamins C and E. Therefore, if a person must smoke, he or she may wish to take vitamin C and E supplements. The exact amounts of these vitamins needed to replace those lost through smoking are unknown. Daily intakes of supplementary vitamins and selenium as discussed on page 51 should be adequate.

What is the risk of cancer among nonsmokers who are exposed to tobacco smoke? Some human studies suggest that a significant increase in lung cancer risk occurs among nonsmoking spouses of smokers. This risk is about two times higher than that found among nonsmoking couples. Furthermore, it has been reported that the smoking behavior of mothers, but not of fathers, influences the lung cancer risk of their children. Although more data are needed to substantiate these findings, nonsmokers should avoid surroundings with high levels of tobacco smoke. It is encouraging to note that smoking is now prohibited in many public places around the United States.

Are heavy drinkers more likely to get cancer? About two thirds of American adults consume alcohol, and about 17 percent of these are considered heavy drinkers. The average yearly consumption of alcohol in the United States is about 3 gallons per person.

There are no data to suggest that moderate consumption of alcohol alone increases the risk of cancer. However, there have been some reports that frequent drinking of wine or beer prepared in certain regions of the world (outside the United States) is associated with an increased risk of cancer of the esophagus, colon and rectum. This is possibly because of impurities in the wine or beer, which may be carcinogenic.

Among alcohol abusers (those who drink heavily daily or most of the days of the week), the risk of not only esophageal cancer, but also cancer of the mouth, head and neck, lip, liver, stomach, colon, rectum and lung is markedly increased. Excessive consumption of alcohol also enhances the cancer-causing effects of smoking. The combined effects of alcohol and smoking on cancer risk are about 2.5 times greater than those produced by alcohol or smoking alone.

It has been suggested that excessive consumption of alcohol may increase the risk of cancer in the following ways:

(a) Alcohol contains small amounts of cancer-causing impurities.

(b) Cancer-causing substances are present in our diet and environment, and they are also formed in the intestine. Alcohol increases their solubility and hence the degree to which they may be absorbed by the body. This in turn may increase the risk of cancer.

(c) Some agents do not act as cancer-causing substances until they are converted to an active form. Alcohol may facilitate the conversion.

(d) Alcohol suppresses the body's immune defense system against cancer.

(e) Alcohol may cause nutritional deficiencies, thereby increasing the risk of cancer. Excessive alcohol may cause a deficiency in proteins, vitamins A, C and E, folic acid, thiamine (B$_1$), pyridoxine (B$_6$) and certain minerals such as magnesium, zinc, iron, copper and molybdenum. Deficiencies in vitamins A, C and E may play an important role in increasing the risk of cancer induced by alcohol.

Thus, to reduce the risk of cancer of the upper intestinal tract, mouth and lung, one should avoid excessive alcohol consumption. Those who consume moderate amounts of alcohol should not smoke at the same time, and should ensure through diet and nutritional supplements that body levels of vitamins A, C and E do not decrease.

Does excessive coffee or tea consumption increase the risk of cancer? Research has shown that caffeinated and decaffeinated coffee contains substances which, at high concentrations, are mutagenic* (produce genetic changes). These results suggest that substances other than caffeine are responsible for changes in the genetic materials. Similarly, some indirect human studies also indicate that excessive consumption of either caffeinated or decaffeinated coffee is associated with an increased risk of bladder, pancreas, and stomach cancer; however, other studies have not confirmed these results. It has been suggested that readily oxidized phenolic compounds which are normally present in coffee facilitate the formation of nitrosamine from nitrite and amines in the stomach. Thus, it appears that if large amounts of nitrosamines are formed in the stomach because of an excessive consumption of coffee, the risk of certain cancers, especially stomach and pancreas cancer, may be increased. Again, caffeine alone does not seem to be associated with an increased risk of cancer. This finding is further supported by the fact that animal studies have so far failed to show that caffeine by itself produces cancer.

---

*Alterations in genetic materials cause mutations which in most cases are not expressed. Examples of expressed mutations include hemophilia, color blindness, and Huntington's chorea. Substances which cause mutations are said to be mutagenic.

A recent study from England has reported that heavy tea consumption increases the risk of cancer of the pancreas. The cancer-causing substances in the tea have not been identified. One of the factors could be caffeine.

It should be pointed out that caffeine is known to cause genetic changes, as well as to reduce the capacity of cells to repair damage produced by agents such as radiation and chemicals. Therefore, it appears that excessive caffeine may enhance the effect of cancer-causing substances so that it acts as a tumor promoter. Further studies are needed to define the role of excessive consumption of coffee, tea, and caffeine in the development of cancer in human beings.

SOME ENVIRONMENTAL AGENTS KNOWN TO CAUSE CANCER

Ionizing Radiation (X Rays and Gamma Rays)

Ionizing radiation is commonly used to diagnose human diseases and to treat cancer. However, it is now well established that such radiation may also cause cancer.

The minimum dose (single and whole-body) needed to induce leukemia in adults is about 20 rad (radiation absorbed dose) (1 rad is equal to the radiation exposure of approximately 33 chest X-ray films). It has been estimated, however, that in human fetuses any amount of radiation may induce leukemia. Repeated exposure to smaller doses of radiation is more likely to produce leukemia than a large single dose. Most leukemias appear within 10 years from the time of radiation exposure.

The minimum dose of radiation needed to produce breast cancer is about 1 rad. Breast tissue is more sensitive to radiation during pregnancy. The minimum time interval between exposure to radiation and cancer development is about 5 years, and the maximum time interval is about 30 years.

The minimum dose of radiation needed to produce thyroid

cancer is about 7 rad. Women are approximately two times more sensitive than men, and Jewish women may be about 17 times more sensitive than non-Jewish women. The reasons for these differences are unknown at this time. The time interval between exposure to radiation and cancer development may vary from 10 years to over 35 years.

Doses commonly used in radiation therapy (a total of 3,000–4,000 rad, given at 200 rad/day, 1,000 rad/week) can induce cancer in most organs 10–30 years after the completion of radiation therapy. This aspect is discussed in detail in Chapter 3.

Since there is no radiation dose known to be "safe," continuous efforts must be made to minimize exposure as much as possible. The extent to which these efforts are successful may well affect the whole future of nuclear energy. No one should be exposed to any extra radiation unless it is necessary for his/her health. There is no reason why a person should not ask his/her physician or dentist if an X-ray examination is really necessary.

Some laboratory studies suggest that the combination of X-radiation and chemical carcinogens is nine times more likely to cause cancer than the individual agents alone. X-radiation also increases virus-induced cancer formation.

Ultraviolet (UV) Radiation

Exposure to UV radiation (part of the radiation from the sun; also called nonionizing radiation) is greater for people who reside at higher altitudes and in areas with high sun exposure. Skin cancers such as melanoma can result from exposure to UV radiation. White skin is more prone to develop melanoma than black; however, the progression of melanoma in persons with black skin is much more rapid than in those with white skin. The use of a sun screen (skin lotion) may reduce the effects of UV radiation during sunbathing. Some studies have reported that the combination of UV radiation and X-radiation is 12 times more likely to produce cancer cells than the individual agents. In addition, tumor promoters present in the diet and environment may also increase the risk of UV radiation-induced cancer formation and may be partly responsible for a five-fold increase in melanoma incidence in the sunbelt states of the U.S. It is interesting to note that chemical carcinogens which increased the risk of X-ray induced cancer failed to increase the risk of UV radiation-induced cancer.

The time interval between exposure to UV radiation and the formation of detectable cancer is generally more than 10 years.

Chemotherapeutic Agents

Most of the chemotherapeutic agents which are currently used in the treatment of cancer can also produce cancer in human beings. It takes about 10–30 years before new cancer will appear after chemotherapy.

Compounds

The following compounds and agents are carcinogenic:

Dioxin, a by-product of herbicide and pesticide production, is one of the most toxic substances produced by humans; exposure to only one part per billion is hazardous to human health.

Polyvinyl chloride (PVC), commonly found in packaging materials.

Pesticides, commonly found in meat and nonmeat foods.

Polychlorinated biphenyls (PCBs), commonly found in packaging materials and fish obtained from contaminated rivers.

Diethylstilbestrol (DES), a synthetic female hormone commonly fed to cattle.

Polycyclic aromatic hydrocarbons, commonly present in air pollution and charcoal-broiled meat.
Asbestos, commonly found in certain building materials such as roofing and water pipe insulation.
Aflatoxin, a mold (fungus) found on peanuts and peanut butter if they are not well preserved.
Heavy metals, such as arsenic, cadmium, mercury and lead.

Viruses

Certain viruses have been shown to cause cancer or increase the risk of cancer in human beings. For example, hepatitis B virus may induce liver cancer, and viruses have been associated with some types of human lymphoma (lymph node tumor). It has been reported that viruses may cause AIDS (acquired immune deficiency syndrome). This disease most frequently afflicts male homosexuals, hemophiliacs and illicit drug users. The same viruses may be responsible for Kaposi sarcoma, a type of cancer that often develops in people with AIDS.

In most animal studies, a single cancer-causing agent is tested to determine its carcinogenic potential. However, human beings are chronically exposed to multiple cancer-causing agents at very low doses. Recent experimental studies of animals have shown that a combination of two cancer-causing agents is more effective in producing cancer than the agents alone. These results suggest that the doses of carcinogens needed to produce cancer in human beings may be very low.

Table 3 describes some dietary and lifestyle factors that may be associated with specific cancer types.

TABLE 3

Relationships Between Diet, Lifestyle and Cancer Risk

Probable Causative Agents (Diet and Lifestyle)	Type of Cancer
Excess fat	Prostate, breast, stomach, colon, rectum, pancreas and ovary
Excess protein	Breast, endometrium, prostate colon, rectum, pancreas and kidney
Excess total caloric intake	Most cancer, not related to any particular types
Excess alcohol	Esophagus, mouth, head and neck, lip, stomach, liver, colon and rectum
Smoking	Lung, larynx, mouth and esophagus
Excess alcohol plus smoking	Mouth, larynx, esophagus, and lung
Excess alcohol, smoking and excess coffee	Pancreas, lung, liver, mouth, larynx, and esophagus
Excess coffee, tea	Bladder, pancreas and stomach
Excess saccharine	Bladder
Cadmium from diet, smoking and occupation	Kidney

(Table 3, continued)

Excess zinc	All cancers, especially breast and stomach
Iron deficiency	Stomach and esophagus
Iodine deficiency	Thyroid
Excess smoked meat or fish, excess charcoal-broiled meat, excess pickled products	Stomach
Certain viruses	Liver, certain blood cancers

MAJOR WARNING SIGNALS FOR CANCER

General: Weakness and weight loss, fatigue.

Breast cancer: Persistent lump, blood or blood-stained discharge from nipple, non-healing ulcer.

Lung cancer: Persistent cough, coughing up blood, chest pain.

Cervix cancer: Spotting of blood after intercourse, painful coitus, foul discharge from vagina.

Skin cancer: Increase in size of mole, ulceration of mole, change in color of mole, pain at the site of mole, non-healing and persistent ulcer.

Rectal and colon cancer: Alternate diarrhea and constipation, blood discharge in stool associated with weight loss.

Stomach cancer: Indigestion, vomiting for a prolonged period of time, loss of appetite.

Bone cancer: Prolonged pain in bone without any injury, with or without swelling.

Testis cancer: Persistent firm to hard swelling in testis, usually without pain.

Hodgkin's Disease: Firm and painless enlargement of lymph nodes, fever, excessive sweating, fatigue.

Leukemia: Weakness, loss of appetite, bone and joint pain, fever, lymph node swelling.

HOW TO PROTECT AGAINST CANCER

We can reduce the risk of cancer in two ways. First, we can attempt to eliminate as many cancer-causing agents (tumor initiators and tumor promoters) from the environment and the diet as possible. Second, we can reduce the effectiveness of carcinogens by taking anticarcinogenic substances. The first approach appears simple, but in reality it is the more difficult, since it requires legislation and dramatic alterations in lifestyles and dietary habits. The second approach appears more practical and may be nearly as effective. This approach involves reducing our intake of cancer-causing substances as much as possible, or practical, and increasing our use of specific dietary components which have been demonstrated to reduce the formation and effectiveness of cancer-causing agents.

What are the known dietary anticancer agents? Many laboratory experiments have shown that there are several agents in the diet which may reduce the risk of cancer caused by radiation and a wide range of chemical carcinogens. These specific anticancer nutrients include the following:

Vitamins

Vitamins A, C and E are potent anticancer agents which may reduce the risk of cancer in animals. Although analyses of dietary habits and cancer incidence have shown that these vitamins may also reduce the risk of cancer in human beings, conclusive proof is still lacking. This is primarily because experiments analogous to animal tumor studies have not been performed in human beings. In animals studies, the effect of a single vitamin on the incidence of cancer is evaluated; in human studies the effectiveness of a diet rich in vitamins A, C and E is generally evaluated, rather than the individual vitamins. Thus, it is difficult to compare animal and human studies. Other vitamins such as vitamin B complex (except riboflavin), vitamin D and vitamin K do not appear to prevent cancer in animals or human beings, but they are necessary for many body functions. Some animal studies have shown that supplemental riboflavin reduces the risk of chemical-induced liver and skin cancer. Deficiency of riboflavin enhances the growth of chemical-induced skin cancer. The relevance of these observations for human cancer is unknown.

Protease Inhibitors

Protease inhibitors are found in soybeans. They are substances that inhibit the activities of cellular enzymes called proteases, which destroy proteins in cells. Some laboratory experiments suggest that adding protease inhibitors, such as antipain substances, blocks cancer formation by X rays and also the action of tumor promoters. The significance of protease inhibitors in reducing the risk of cancer in human beings remains to be evaluated.

Minerals

Among minerals, selenium appears to be a very potent anticancer agent for animal tumors. Analyses of dietary intake of selenium and cancer incidence have shown that it may also reduce the risk of cancer in human beings.

Other Dietary Factors

Among other dietary factors, fiber appears to be most important in reducing the risk of cancer, especially of colon and rectal cancer.

HOW VITAMINS CAN PREVENT CANCER

Vitamins A, C and E may reduce the incidence of cancer in multiple ways, some of which are described below:

Vitamins can act as antioxidants: Vitamin A (beta-carotene, retinol, retinoic acid, but not retinyl palmitate or retinyl acetate), vitamin E (alpha-tocopherol, but not alpha-tocopheryl acetate, alpha-tocopheryl succinate or alpha-tocopheryl nicotinate), and vitamin C (ascorbic acid or sodium ascorbate) act as antioxidants; that is, they destroy free radicals, a harmful chemical species that is formed normally in the body. Many cancer-causing agents affect normal cells by generating free radicals. Thus, higher levels of these vitamins within or outside cells may protect them from the damaging effects of free radicals.

Vitamins can inhibit cancer-causing substances: Vitamins C and E, but not vitamin A, may prevent the formation and reduce the levels of certain cancer-causing substances in the intestinal tract. For example, nitrites are commonly used to preserve meat and are present in bacon, sausage, hot dogs, and cured meat. Nitrites by themselves do not cause cancer, but they can combine with amines in the stomach to form nitrosamines.

NITRITE + AMINE = NITROSAMINE

Nitrosamines are among the most potent cancer-causing agents for both animals and human beings. They are very soluble in water and therefore can be readily absorbed and distributed to all the tissues in the body. The presence of vitamin C or vitamin E (alpha-tocopherol) in the stomach may prevent the formation or reduce the levels of nitrosamines.

NITRITE + AMINE + VITAMIN C OR
VITAMIN E = LITTLE OR NO NITROSAMINE

Thus, taking vitamin C or vitamin E just before eating food containing nitrites may reduce or prevent the formation of nitrosamines in the stomach. The amounts of vitamin C or vitamin E needed depend upon the amounts of nitrites to be consumed. At this time it is impossible to determine precisely the amounts of vitamin C or vitamin E needed to reduce the formation of nitrosamines. However, one can estimate that for an average meal containing nitrites, taking 200 milligrams of vitamin C and 50 I.U. of alpha-tocopherol immediately before eating may be adequate.

In addition to nitrosamines, many other mutagenic substances (agents which cause genetic changes that may or may not lead to cancer) are formed in the intestinal tract. Many mutations (changes in genetic materials) precede cancer formation. It has been shown that the levels of mutagenic substances in the feces are higher for persons who are meat eaters than for those who are vegetarians. The presence of higher levels of fecal mutagenic substances may increase the risk of cancer. This hypothesis is supported by the fact that the incidence of cancer among Seventh Day Adventists who are vegetarians is much less than for those who eat meat. It has been reported that taking vitamin C or vitamin E reduces the levels of mutagenic substances in the feces. Furthermore, reports indicate that taking both vitamins C and E is more effective than taking either individually. In a current human trial, 400 milligrams of vitamin C and 400 I.U. of alpha-tocopherol are being used by persons who have a high risk of developing polyps, a precursor of colon cancer. The full results of this trial are unavailable at this time, so it is difficult to estimate the amounts of vitamins needed; however, doses of 250 milligrams of vitamin C and 100 I.U. of alpha-tocopherol may be adequate to reduce the levels of mutagenic substances in the intestine.

In addition, many chemicals are not carcinogenic until they are converted to an active form in the body. In some cases vitamins A, C and E can prevent the conversion of inactive forms of such cancer-causing substances to active forms.

Vitamins can reduce the action of cancer-causing agents: Many experimental studies suggest that vitamins A, C and E may inhibit the cancer-causing action of tumor promoters as well as tumor initiators. In order for such inhibition to occur, high levels of vitamins A, C and E must be maintained in the cells; the optimal doses are unknown. Recommended doses and dose schedules of vitamins for cancer prevention are described on page 51.

Vitamins can change newly formed or established cancer cells back to normal cells: Some recent laboratory experiments suggest that vitamins A, C and E may convert newly formed or well established cancer cells to normal cells. For example, vitamin C has been shown to reverse new chemically induced cancer cells to normal cells. Vitamin C does not have this effect on well established cancer cells. However, vitamin A has been shown to transform some well established cancer cells to cells resembling normal cells. Some tumors such as lung cancer, prostate cancer, colon cancer and neuroblastoma (a tumor of embryonic nerve cells) respond to vitamin A in the above manner. Similarly, alpha-tocopheryl succinate also transforms some established cancer cells such as melanoma (a form of skin cancer) to normal cells. It also permanently stops the growth of some other tumor cells such as glioma tumor, prostate carcinoma, neuroblastoma and leukemia cells. Recent laboratory experiments show that vitamin E alpha-tocopheryl is more potent than other forms of vitamin E (e.g., alpha-tocopheryl acetate and alpha-tocopheryl) in reducing the growth of cancer cells and enabling them to become more like normal cells.

The exact amounts of vitamins needed to reverse cancer cells to normal cells are not known for human beings; however, the doses and dose schedules described on page 51 may be adequate for this mechanism.

Vitamins can stimulate the body's immune defense system against cancer: Vitamins A, C and E have been shown to stimulate the body's defense system, which in turn may kill newly formed cancer cells, or the remaining few established cancer cells, in patients who are in a state of remission. The amounts needed to achieve these effects are unknown. However, some studies have shown that vitamin C (up to 4 grams per day), vitamin E alpha-tocopherol (1,200 I.U. orally per day) and vitamin A (12,000 I.U. orally per day) stimulate the human body's immune defense system.

The vitamin mechanisms described above are relevant to cancer prevention. These mechanisms of action of vitamins are now being studied in human beings. In a large human trial involving more than 5,000 subjects in England, it was found that low blood levels of vitamin E were associated with an increased risk of breast cancer. The risk was five times higher among those women who have lowest levels of blood vitamin E, than in those who have highest blood levels of vitamin E. Higher blood levels of beta-carotene and vitamin A also appear to have protective value. To demonstrate the involvement of vitamins in the prevention of human cancer, we must show that an increased intake of supplementary vitamin A, vitamin C, vitamin E, or all three, reduces the risk of cancer among high risk human populations. Some high risk populations are smokers (lung cancer), asbestos workers (lung cancer), and persons with polyps (colon cancer). Only such human studies can be considered analogous to animal experiments in which large amounts of supplemental vitamins in the diet have reduced the risk of chemically induced tumors. Several such human studies are currently in progress, and others are being planned. A definitive answer regarding the role of vitamins A, C and E in the prevention of human cancer will come from these studies, but it will be 40 to 50 years before complete data become available. Thus, interim dietary and supplementary nutrition guidelines should be considered **tentative** and open to revision as new scientific results on human beings become available. (When estimating doses of vitamins to be taken on a regular basis, one must also be aware of dose ranges within which these vitamins do not produce any toxic effects in human beings).

Most of the above descriptions of vitamin mechanisms are based on animal studies. Sometimes animal studies are criticized because the doses of carcinogens that produce tumors in animals are very high and since human beings generally are not exposed to such high doses, animal studies are not relevant. This type of criticism may not be valid. It should always be remembered that human beings are exposed to low doses of many cancer-causing agents every day. In experiments, animals are exposed to only one cancer-causing agent, and therefore high doses of chemicals are needed for cancer to develop. Thus it seems reasonable to believe that doses needed to produce cancer in human beings would be much smaller than those needed for animals. It is true that animal data cannot be directly extrapolated to human beings, but such data do suggest that the same cancer-causing agents will in most instances produce cancer in human beings as well.

VITAMIN NUTRITION

What are some rich dietary sources of vitamins?

Vitamin A

Vegetables: Beet greens, broccoli, carrots, pumpkins, spinach, sweet potatoes, cabbage, lettuce, yellow corn

Fruits: Cantaloupe, apricots, mangoes
Animal Products: Liver, eggs, milk
For Retinol: Eggs are the best source.
For Beta-carotene: Yellow vegetables and fruits, cabbage, spinach, and lettuce are excellent sources.

Vitamin C

Vegetables: Brussels sprouts, cauliflower, peas, cabbage, green peppers
Fruits: Oranges, lemons, limes, pineapples, raspberries, strawberries, grapefruit

Vitamin E

Vegetables: Spinach, parsley, mustard greens, turnip leaves, sweet potatoes, vegetable oils
Fruits and Nuts: Apple skins, tomatoes, cucumbers, almonds
Animal Products: Fish

What forms of synthesized vitamins are available?

Vitamin A

Forms: Beta-carotene, retinyl acetate, retinol and retinyl palmitate. Beta-carotene is converted to retinol in the wall of the intestines, and retinyl acetate is converted to retinol in both the lumen and the wall of the intestine.
In Blood: Primarily retinol and some carotenoids.
In Tissues: Primarily retinoic acid; stored in the liver as retinyl palmitate.
Solubility: Soluble in lipids and alcohol but not in water.

Vitamin A should be taken both as beta-carotene and as retinol, retinyl acetate or retinyl palmitate. Laboratory experiments suggest that solvents of some vitamin A preparations are very toxic. Thus, the use of such solvents should be avoided. A vitamin A preparation in a gelatin capsule containing water and glycerine or oil may be recommended.

Vitamin C

Forms: Vitamin C is sold commercially as ascorbic acid, sodium ascorbate (1 gram of vitamin C contains 124 milligrams of sodium), sodium ascorbate—minimum sodium (1 gram of vitamin C contains 62 milligrams of sodium), calcium ascorbate, timed-release capsules containing ascorbic acid, and capsules containing ascorbic acid and certain minerals.

In Blood and Tissues: Primarily ascorbic acid.

Solubility: Both sodium ascorbate and calcium ascorbate are easily dissolved in water.

If one has no signs of hypertension or hyperacidity, sodium ascorbate with minimum sodium is acceptable. If hypertension is present, ascorbic acid or calcium ascorbate may be recommended. If stomach hyperacidity is present, sodium ascorbate or calcium ascorbate may be recommended.

Vitamin E

Forms: Synthetic forms are referred to as dl-forms; natural forms are referred to as d-forms. The common commercial form of vitamin E is d- or dl-alpha-tocopherol or alpha-tocopherol. Other forms of vitamin E are d- or dl-alpha-tocopheryl acetate, alpha-tocopheryl succinate, and alpha-tocopheryl nicotinate. These forms of vitamin E are converted to alpha-tocopherol in the lumen and wall of the intestine.

In Blood and Tissue: Primarily alpha-tocopherol.

Solubility: Soluble in lipids and alcohol, but not in water.

Laboratory experiments have shown that the solvents of some vitamin E preparations are toxic. Therefore, the use of such solvents should be avoided. A vitamin E preparation in a gelatin capsule containing water and glycerine or oil is recommended. Vitamin E should be taken both as alpha-tocopherol and alpha-tocopheryl acetate or alpha-tocopheryl succinate.

How to store vitamins

Vitamin A

Crystal forms of retinol and retinoic may be stored in the cold, away from light, for several months. Other forms of vitamin A can also be stored in the cold.

Vitamin C

Vitamin C should not be stored in solution form because it is easily destroyed. Crystal or tablet forms of vitamin C can be stored at room temperature, away from light, for several months.

Vitamin E

Alpha-tocopherol can be stored in the cold, away from light, whereas vitamin E acetate and vitamin E succinate can be stored at room temperature or in the cold for several months.

Can vitamins be destroyed during storage?

Vitamin A

No form of vitamin A in solution will degrade significantly at room temperature, at least for several months. However, retinoic acid and retinol (solution or powder) are rapidly destroyed when they are exposed to light. Domestic cooking does not destroy retinol and beta-carotene, but slow heating over a long period of time may reduce their potency. Canning and prolonged cold storage may also reduce vitamin A activity. The vitamin A content of fortified milk powder substantially decreases after two years.

Vitamin C

Vitamin C in solution is destroyed by light, heat and air. Freezing, thawing, and cold storage of solutions of vitamin C reduce its potency. Vitamin C solutions in the presence of air and copper, iron or manganese generate free radicals (harmful chemical species). Thus, the mixing of vitamin C with any of these minerals should be avoided. The vitamin C content of fortified milk powder is unaffected over a two year period.

Vitamin E

Vitamin E in solution is easily destroyed, where-as vitamin E acetate and vitamin E succinate solutions are not. Destruction of vitamin E increases in the presence of light, oxygen and trace metals such as iron and copper. Food processing, frying, freezing and drying quickly destroy vitamin E. The vitamin E content of fortified milk powder is unaffected over a two year period.

WHY WE NEED VITAMIN SUPPLEMENTS

Does the human body make its own vitamins? Human beings do not make their own vitamins A, C, and E. We depend on fresh fruits, vegetables, fish, meat, and dairy products, as well as vitamin supplements, for these essential nutrients.

Vitamin A—primarily from fresh fruits and vegetables, liver and eggs.
Vitamin C—primarily from fresh fruits and vegetables.
Vitamin E—primarily from fresh fruits and vegetables and fish.

When we take vitamins, how much does the body absorb?

Vitamin A

Only about 10–20 percent of ingested vitamin A is absorbed from the small intestine. It is characteristic of normal cells that they do not pick up more than they need to function. Liver cells are an exception. Retinol is absorbed more readily than beta-carotene. Beta-carotene and retinyl acetate are converted to retinol in the wall of the intestine. Retinol is further converted to retinoic acid in cells; however, most of the body's vitamin A is stored in the liver as retinyl palmitate.

Since the maximum level of retinol in blood appears 3–6 hours after ingestion of vitamin A and drops to a basal level in about 10–12 hours, it should be taken twice a day (once in the morning and once in the evening) to maintain higher levels.

Vitamin C

The amount of absorption of ingested vitamin C varies from 20–80 percent, depending upon the dose. If one consumes 200–500 milligrams, only 50 percent (100–250 milligrams) will be absorbed from the intestine. If one takes more than the above doses, absorption of vitamin C is further reduced. On this basis, one should not take more than 500 milligrams per dose. It should be pointed out that in order to reduce the formation of cancer-causing substances in the stomach and intestine, certain amounts of unabsorbed vitamin C may be useful. Once absorbed, vitamin C is rapidly distributed throughout the body. As with vitamin A, normal cells do not pick up more vitamin C than they need to function.

Since vitamin C is rapidly degraded in the body, the maintenance of effective blood levels may require taking vitamin C at least four times a day.

Vitamin E

Vitamin E can be taken as alpha-tocopherol, vitamin E acetate or vitamin E succinate. Vitamin E acetate and succinate are converted to vitamin E in the lumen of the intestine prior to being absorbed. About 20 percent of ingested vitamin E is absorbed from the small intestine in the form of vitamin E and is rapidly distributed throughout the body. As with vitamins A and C, normal cells do not pick up greater amounts of vitamin E than they need.

Since the maximum levels of vitamin E in the blood appear 4–6 hours after vitamin E is ingested and drop to a basal level in about 12 hours, the maintenance of higher blood levels of vitamin E requires taking it twice a day (morning and evening).

Which vitamins should we take, how much, and how often? At this time, the doses of vitamins for the greatest benefit to human health or for maximum reduction of cancer risk are unknown. Recommended Daily Allowances (RDA) for vitamins and other nutrients are listed in Tables 4–7.

At present there are two opinions regarding the importance of these current RDA values. One group of scientists believes that RDA values are adequate for maintaining good human health and that larger amounts of vitamins may be harmful. Another group of scientists believes that the current RDA values for vitamins are enough to prevent deficiency, but that larger amounts may be needed to maintain good health and especially to prevent cancer. Experimental results from animal studies support the view that higher doses are needed for cancer prevention.

TABLE 4

Recommended Daily Allowances (RDA) for Vitamins

Vitamins	RDA
VITAMIN A	
Adult male	5,000 I.U.
Adult female	4,000 I.U.
Pregnancy	5,000 I.U.
VITAMIN C	
Adult male	60 mg.
Adult female	60 mg.
Pregnancy	80 mg.
Lactation	100 mg.
VITAMIN E	
Adult male	15 I.U.
Adult female	15 I.U.
Pregnancy and lactation	18 I.U.
VITAMIN D	
Adult male	200–300 I.U.
Adult female	200–300 I.U.
Pregnancy and lactation	400 I.U.
VITAMIN K	
Adults	No specific requirements
THIAMINE	
Adults	1 mg.
Pregnancy	1.4 mg.
Lactation	1.5 mg.

(Table 4, continued)

RIBOFLAVIN	
Adults	1.2 mg.
Pregnancy	1.5 mg.
Lactation	1.7 mg.

NIACIN	
Adults	6.5 mg.
Pregnancy	7.5 mg.
Lactation	8.5 mg.

VITAMIN B$_6$	
Adults	Up to 2 mg.
Pregnancy	2.6 mg.
Lactation	2.5 mg.

FOLACIN	
Adults	400 μg.
Pregnancy	800 μg.
Lactation	500 μg.

VITAMIN B$_{12}$	
Adults	3 μg.
Pregnancy and lactation	4 μg.

mg. = *milligram*
μg. = *microgram*
I.U. = *International Unit*

TABLE 5

Recommended Daily Allowances (RDA) for Trace Metals

Trace Metals	RDA
IRON	
Adult male	10 mg.
Adult female	18 mg.
Pregnancy	30-60 mg.
ZINC	
Adult male	15 mg.
Adult female	15 mg.
Pregnancy	20 mg.
Lactation	25 mg.
IODINE	
Adult male	150 μg.
Adult female	150 μg.
Pregnancy	175 μg.
Lactation	200 μg.
COPPER	
Adults	2–3 mg.
MANGANESE	
Adults	2.5–5 mg.
FLUORIDE	
Adults	1.5–4 mg.
CHROMIUM	
Adults	500–200 μg.
MOLYBDENUM	
Adults	0.15–0.5 mg.
SELENIUM	
Adults	50–200 μg.

TABLE 6

Recommended Daily Allowances (RDA) for Minerals

Minerals	RDA
CALCIUM	
Adults	800 mg.
Pregnancy and lactation	1200 mg.
PHOSPHORUS	
Adults	800 mg.
MAGNESIUM	
Adult male	350 mg.
Adult female	300 mg.
Pregnancy and lactation	450 mg.

TABLE 7

Recommended Daily Allowances (RDA) for Nutrients

Nutrients	RDA
CARBOHYDRATE and FIBER	No specific requirements
FAT	No specific requirements, 15–25 grams may be adequate.
PROTEINS	0.8 milligram per kilogram of body weight; or 60 grams for a 75 kilogram (165 lb.) person. Need increases during pregnancy, lactation, work, stress and aging.

Even though we do not have sufficient scientific information regarding doses of vitamins needed to reduce the risk of cancer in human beings, **interim** guidelines for taking supplemental vitamins have been developed for the following reasons:

1. Adequate animal data are already available.
2. It will be 40 to 50 years before adequate human data become available. Many of us cannot wait that long.
3. Without interim guidelines it is left to the individual to assess his/her own needs for dietary and supplemental vitamins. Some studies have estimated that 40 percent of all Americans take supplemental vitamins and other nutrients on a regular basis. When one talks with some of these people, it become apparent that many are consuming nutrients in amounts which may not be helpful and may even be harmful.

INTERIM GUIDELINES FOR SUPPLEMENTAL VITAMINS

The following doses and dose schedules of vitamins A, C and E are based on animal and human studies, are unlikely to produce any major side effects in the average normal adult, and may reduce the risk of cancer.

Vitamin A

A total of 7,500 I.U. per day, taken orally, divided into two doses, once in the morning and once in the evening (each dose containing 2,500 I.U. of retinol or retinyl acetate and 1,250 I.U. of beta-carotene).

The average dietary consumption of vitamin A by Americans is about 2,500 I.U. per day. It is unlikely that a total daily consumption of 10,000 I.U. (diet plus supplement) will produce any side effects.

The reason for taking vitamin A twice a day is that the blood levels of vitamin A reach a maximum level in 3–6 hours and drop to an original level 10–12 hours after ingestion. Thus, in order to maintain sustained high levels of vitamin A in the blood an oral intake of vitamin A twice a day is needed.

Both beta-carotene and retinol, or retinyl acetate, have been included in the supplemental vitamin recommendations because beta-carotene, in addition to being a precursor of retinol, appears to have some other actions of its own.

Vitamin C

A total of 1 gram per day, taken orally, divided into four doses (each dose containing 250 milligrams of vitamin C), or divided into two doses (each dose containing 500 milligrams of vitamin C in a timed-release capsule).

The average dietary consumption of vitamin C by Americans is about 20 to 40 milligrams per day. It is unlikely that a total daily intake of 1 gram plus 20 to 40 milligrams of dietary vitamin C will produce any side effects.

The reason for taking vitamin C at least four times a day, or twice a day in timed-release capsules, is that the blood levels of vitamin C rise rapidly after its ingestion and drop to an original level 4–6 hours later. Thus, in order to maintain a sustained high level of vitamin C in the blood, a frequent oral intake of vitamin C is needed.

Vitamin E

A total of 200 I.U. per day, taken orally, divided into two doses, one in the morning and one in the evening (each dose containing 50 I.U. of vitamin E acetate or succinate and 50 I.U. of alpha-tocopherol).

The average dietary consumption of vitamin E by Americans is about 10–20 I.U. per day. It seems unlikely that a total daily intake of 210–220 I.U. of vitamin E (diet plus supplement) will produce any side effects.

The reason for taking vitamin E twice a day is that the blood level of vitamin E reach a maximum level about 4–6 hours after ingestion. Thus, in order to maintain sustained high levels of vitamin E in the blood, an oral intake of vitamin E twice a day is needed.

Both vitamin E alpha-tocopherol and vitamin E acetate or vitamin E succinate have been included because vitamin E acetate and vitamin E succinate cannot act as antioxidants until they are converted to the vitamin E alpha-tocopherol form. Thus, the presence of vitamin E alpha-tocopherol in the stomach is necessary in order to block carcinogenic events such as the formation of nitrosamines.

Riboflavin

At this time, there are no sufficient data from animals or human beings to recommend riboflavin supplements. No cases of riboflavin toxicity in animals or human beings have been reported.

Do we need supplementary vitamins if we have a balanced diet? For nutrition, no; for cancer prevention, probably yes.

It would be very difficult for anyone to eat fresh fruits and vegetables daily in the amounts and at frequencies which would maintain sustained high levels of vitamins A, C and E in the blood; therefore, consumption of supplemental vitamins is essential, in addition to eating a balanced diet.

One of the advantages of the supplemental vitamins is that one can take them at the most appropriate time, especially just before eating food containing nitrites or other cancer-causing substances, in order to prevent the formation of cancer-causing agents and reduce their carcinogenic effects.

Some scientists believe that a balanced diet is sufficient to maintain good health and prevent disease. However, recent studies suggest that all naturally occuring foods have toxic substances as well as protective substances inherent in their constitution; therefore, a balanced diet alone may not be sufficient for disease prevention. While it is true that a balanced diet is better than junk food and that it will prevent vitamin deficiency, the main problem with the concept of a balanced diet is that it is very general, and the interpretation of this concept may vary markedly from one individual to another. Some persons may believe that a daily intake of one apple, one carrot, one orange, some fresh vegetables, meat and carbohydrates constitutes a balanced diet, whereas others may believe that a believe that a balanced diet should contain five times as much fresh produce. Thus, the concept that a balanced diet is adequate for maximum protection against cancer may not be correct.

Even if a balanced diet is defined more precisely, the same balanced diet cannot be applied to all the regions of the world because dietary and environmental levels of precursors* of cancer-causing substances, tumor promoters, and tumor initiators vary markedly from one region to another. Thus, supplemental vitamins may be necessary to reduce the risk of cancer.

With respect to cancer prevention, it is important to ingest certain vitamins at the right time; otherwise their possible

---

*Some chemicals do not cause cancer until they are converted to a cancer-causing form. These chemicals are called precursors.

effectiveness against cancer may be minimized. For example, vitamins C and E, if taken immediately before eating food containing nitrites, may reduce the formation of nitrosamines in the stomach. Taking these vitamins a few hours after such a meal may not effectively interfere with this stage of carcinogenesis. Furthermore, it has been demonstrated that levels of fecal mutagens (a possible source of cancer) in persons who regularly eat meat are much higher than in those who are vegetarians. Ingestion of vitamin C and vitamin E has been shown to reduce the levels of mutagens in the feces. Therefore, it is important that these vitamins be taken before or right after eating meat. Taking these vitamins several hours after such a meal may not be very effective.

In addition, when one travels or vacations away from home, the quantities of fresh fruits and vegetables needed to provide sufficient vitamins may not be available. Thus, supplemental vitamins are also needed under these conditions.

It may not be the absolute amounts of vitamins which are important in cancer prevention. Instead, it may be the relative levels of cancer-causing substances present in the diet and the environment and anticancer substances such as vitamins and selenium in the body that are crucial in determining the potential for cancer. Consequently, increased consumption of cancer-causing substances via diet and environment would require a proportional increase in available anticancer substances.

RISKS OF TAKING VITAMINS

Vitamin A

Liver toxicity and skin reactions have been noted after oral ingestion of 50,000 I.U. per day of vitamin A over a long period of time. Some of these changes are reversible after the practice is discontinued. Dosages of 20,000 I.U. of vitamin A or less, taken orally and divided into two doses per day, are unlikely to produce any major toxic effects in an average normal adult.

Vitamin C

In most healthy persons, doses of vitamin C up to 10 grams per day taken orally do not produce any detectable toxic effects. However, in certain diseases involving iron metabolism (hemochromatosis), copper metabolism (Wilson's disease), and excessive exposure to manganese (Parkinsonian-like syndrome), an excessive consumption of vitamin C may be harmful, because vitamin C in combination with iron, copper or manganese, in the presence of oxygen, generates free radicals (harmful chemical species). According to many studies, dosages up to one gram of vitamin C, taken orally and divided into 4 doses per day, are unlikely to cause any serious side effects in an average normal adult.

Vitamin E

In a large human trial involving 9,000 adults, a daily oral intake of 3,000 I.U. per day of vitamin E acetate for 11 years did not produce any detectable major side effects; however, isolated cases of fatigue, skin reactions and upset stomach have been reported after ingestion of high doses (above 1,000 I.U. daily) of vitamin E for a prolonged period of time. According to many studies, dosages up to 400 I.U. of vitamin E taken orally, divided into two doses per day, are unlikely to produce any major toxic effects in an average normal adult.

DIETARY FIBER AND
REDUCED CANCER RISK

Some human and animal studies suggest that a diet containing high levels of fiber may reduce the risk of certain cancers, especially large bowel cancer (colon and rectal). The incidence of these cancers is virtually absent among people of northwest India (Punjabi) who eat a diet rich in roughage, cellulose, vegetables, fiber and yogurt, in comparison with South Indians who do not eat such foods. Also, as noted previously, the incidence of cancer in general is much lower among Seventh Day Adventists, who are vegetarians. It is believed that a diet high in fiber results in regular bowel movements, which reduce the body's contact time with cancer-causing substances normally formed in the intestine and intestinal tissue. This may reduce the absorption of carcinogens and thereby reduce the risk of cancer. Further human studies are needed before the ability of fiber to help prevent cancer of the large bowel is confirmed beyond doubt.

Excessive dietary fiber may reduce the absorption of minerals, so supplemental amounts of fiber are not recommended. An adequate amount of fiber can be obtained from fresh fruits and vegetables and whole-grain cereals.

SELENIUM

How does selenium prevent cancer? Small amounts of selenium are absolutely essential for good health, and among minerals only selenium has been shown to have a role in cancer prevention. The very limited data for human beings tend to confirm the anticancer effects of selenium.

Like vitamin E, selenium acts as an antioxidant and strengthens the body's immune defense system. Thus, many of the effects that are produced by vitamin E deficiency can be reversed or prevented by selenium. Some laboratory experiments have suggested that the combination of vitamin E and selenium is more effective in preventing cancer than either of them alone.

Metals that block the action of selenium: Certain metals such as lead, cadmium, arsenic, mercury and silver block the action of selenium.

It is commonly believed that high doses of zinc are very good for maintaining health, but this may not be true with respect to cancer prevention. Recent laboratory experiments have shown that high doses of zinc block the action of selenium. Therefore, one has to be careful about taking excessive amounts of zinc (over 20 milligrams total per day from diet and supplements) while taking selenium.

Nutrients that increase selenium requirements: Protein-rich and unsaturated fat-rich diets have been shown to increase the selenium requirements of the body.

These studies suggest that to get the greatest cancer preventing benefits of selenium, a diet low in those metals that block the action of selenium and that provides adequate but not excessive amounts of zinc, protein and unsaturated fats should be considered.

How to select supplementary selenium: Commercial preparations of selenium include inorganic selenium (sodium selenite) and various organic compounds of selenium. It has been reported that sodium selenite is not absorbed adequately, whereas organic selenium, including yeast-selenium, is absorbed very well. For this reason, yeast-selenium is considered best for human consumption.

How much selenium should one take and how often? The optimal doses of selenium for health benefits are unknown. The current average dietary intake of selenium is about 125–150 micrograms per day. Based on 0.1 microgram of selenium per gram of diet, the RDA value of selenium for adults is 50–200 micrograms per day. It has been reported that selenium dosages of about 250–300 micrograms per day (diet and supplements) would be helpful in preventing cancer. If an average person consumes 125–150 micrograms of selenium per day, an additional supplemental amount of 100 micrograms per day is unlikely to produce any major side effects.

Risks of taking selenium: Animal studies suggest that 2–3 micrograms per gram of diet (20–30 times the human RDA) per day may produce toxic side effects.

TABLE 8

Summary of the Actions of Vitamins and Selenium in Cancer Prevention

Nutrients	Preventive Action
Vitamin C and vitamin E (alpha-tocopherol)	Block the formation of cancer-causing agents.
	Block the conversion of some cancer-causing agents to an active form.
Vitamin A (retinol and beta-carotene), vitamin C, vitamin E (alpha-tocopherol) and selenium	Block the action of tumor-causing agents (initiators and promoters).
Vitamins A, C and E	Reverse newly formed cancer cells back to normal cells.
Vitamins A, C, E and selenium	Kill newly formed cancer cells in the body by stimulating the body's immune defense system.

NUTRIENTS THAT MAY INCREASE
THE RISK OF CANCER

Excessive total fat. Both human studies and animal experiments suggest that increasing the intake of total fat increases the risk of certain cancers, particularly breast and colon cancer, and conversely, that lowering fat intake reduces the risk of these cancers. Data from animal studies suggest that when total fat intake is low, polyunsaturated fats are more likely to cause cancer than saturated fats. However, the relevance of this observation for human beings is not clear at this time. In addition, specific components of fat responsible for enhanced carcinogenesis have not been identified, although some studies have indicated that excessive cholesterol consumption may increase the risk of cancer. Extensive human studies are needed to define the role of excessive cholesterol in carcinogenesis.

The exact reasons for the effects of a high fat diet on cancer risk are unknown. However, some recent laboratory experiments have reported that the production of prostaglandin E2 (PGE2), a chemical which is normally produced by the body, is markedly increased in animals which are fed a high fat diet. High levels of PGE2 have been shown to impair the body's immune defense system. Therefore, the increased risk of cancer brought about by a high fat diet may be due to the suppression of the body's defense system against cancer.

It has also been reported that high doses of vitamin E reduce the production of PGE2 and consequently that high doses of vitamin E may block the harmful effects of excessive fat consumption. This does not mean that one should continue eating a high fat diet and take large amounts of vitamin E. Such practices may be very harmful because a high fat diet may increase the risk of heart attack.

Excessive protein. Based on limited laboratory and human studies, it appears that an excessive intake of protein may be associated with an increased risk of cancer of the breast, endometrium, prostate, colon, rectum, pancreas and kidney. A lower protein intake seems to reduce the risk of cancer. Although animal studies suggest a specific role for protein in carcinogenesis, human studies are not convincing. Since the Western diet contains significant amounts of meat, a rich source of both protein and fat, it is difficult to determine an independent role for protein in human carcinogenesis at this time. However, the fact that animal experiments show that high protein intake increases the incidence of chemically induced tumors indicates that proteins may have a similar role in human cancer. Additional studies are needed to substantiate this particular point.

Excessive total calories and excessive carbohydrates. There are some limited studies that suggest that increased total caloric intake may increase the risk of cancer, but the data on both animals and human beings are sparse and indirect. Further studies are needed to answer this question.

There are no scientific data to suggest that an excessive intake of carbohydrates is directly related to the risk of cancer in animals or in human beings. However, excessive consumption of carbohydrates may increase total caloric intake. Additional studies are needed to define the role of carbohydrates in human carcinogenesis.

HOW TO DESIGN YOUR NUTRITION AND LIFESTYLE PROGRAM TO REDUCE THE RISK OF CANCER

Several scientific agencies such as the National Academy of Science, American Cancer Society and the American Institute for Cancer Research have published diet guidelines for reducing cancer risk. These contain very useful information, but no recommendations as yet for supplementary vitamins. The Cancer Research Institute, New York, has also prepared diet guidelines which do contain recommendations for supplementary vitamins and other nutrients. Even though there are no solid human data which suggest that supplemental vitamins A, C and E and selenium are essential for reducing the risk of cancer, there are sufficient animal and limited human studies which indicate that interim guidelines for supplementary vitamins and minerals should also be developed.

Interim guidelines for diet: Increase the consumption of fresh fruits and vegetables. Table 9 describes some vitamin-rich fruits and vegetables that can be eaten for breakfast, lunch and dinner.

INTERIM GUIDELINES FOR SUPPLEMENTARY NUTRITION

Vitamin A

7,500 I.U. per day, taken orally, divided into two doses— once in the morning and once in the evening (each dose containing 2,500 I.U. of retinol or retinyl acetate and 1,250 I.U. of beta-carotene).

Vitamin C

1 gram per day, divided into four doses, each containing 250 milligrams of vitamin C in powder or tablet form, taken orally, four times a day; or divided into two doses, each containing 500 milligrams of vitamin C in a timed-release capsule, taken orally, twice a day.

Vitamin E

200 I.U. per day, divided into two doses, each dose containing 50 I.U. of vitamin E (alpha-tocopherol) and 50 I.U. of vitamin E acetate or succinate, taken orally, twice a day.

Selenium

100 micrograms of yeast-selenium per day, divided into two doses.

INTERIM LIFE STYLE GUIDELINES

1. Reduce consumption of total fat by 30–35 percent (to about two thirds of your current level).
2. Avoid excessive protein and carbohydrate.
3. Avoid excessive zinc.
4. Avoid drinking excessive alcohol, caffeinated or decaffeinated coffee, and tea.
5. Avoid foods with high nitrite content. Whenever eating such foods, take 250 milligrams of vitamin C and 100 I.U. of vitamin E (containing both vitamin E [alpha-tocopherol] and vitamin E acetate or vitamin E succinate) immediately before eating.
6. Avoid eating excessive charcoal-broiled or smoked meat or fish. Whenever such foods are eaten, take 250 milligrams of vitamin C and 100 I.U. of vitamin E (containing both vitamin E [alpha-tocopherol] and vitamin E acetate or vitamin E succinate) before or immediately after eating.
7. DO NOT SMOKE. It you must, take an additional 500 milligrams of vitamin C every day. Do not increase the amounts of vitamin E or vitamin A more than those described above for daily use.

8. Reduce your consumption of pickled fruits and vegetables as much as possible.

At this time, children should not be given supplemental vitamins or selenium in the amounts recommended for an average normal adult. However, the diet and lifestyle guidelines may be equally useful for children.

ADDITIONAL BENEFITS OF FOLLOWING A CANCER PREVENTION PROGRAM

Adapting one's diet, supplementary nutrition and lifestyle for cancer prevention is not limited *only* to cancer protection. Such a program may also be very useful for maintaining sound health, possibly because vitamins protect the body against injurious effects of agents that do not cause cancer. For example, accidental consumption of excess amounts of mercury compounds have produced severe neurological diseases in human beings. Lower doses of mercury compounds may cause behavioral disturbances. Some laboratory experiments suggest that vitamin E reduced the risk of developing neurological diseases when supplemental vitamins were given to animals during exposure to mercury compounds.

Harmful chemical species called free radicals are normally produced in the body. Some of these free radicals are needed to maintain certain vital cell functions. However, if free radicals are produced in excess amounts, either because of genetic defects or through consumption of agents that generate large quantities of free radicals in the body, some vital organs may be permanently damaged. The presence of vitamins A, C and E and selenium in the body in sufficient amounts may protect these organs against the injurious effects of free radicals.

TABLE 9

Interim Dietary Guidelines for Vitamin-Rich Fruits and Vegetables

---

BREAKFAST
(Select one or more from each category)

Vitamin A-rich fruits:
Apricots, mangoes, peaches, cantaloupe

Vitamin C-rich fruits:
Oranges, limes, lemons, pineapple, strawberries, raspberries

Vitamin E-rich fruits:
Apple with skin (also recommended: eggs, milk)

LUNCH
(Select one or more from each category)

Vitamin A-rich vegetables
Asparagus, spinach, carrots, broccoli, corn, pumpkins, cabbage

Vitamin C-rich vegetables:
Brussels sprouts, cauliflower, peas, cabbage, green peppers

Vitamin E-rich vegetables
Spinach, parsley, mustard greens, turnip leaves, sweet potatoes, cucumbers

DINNER
(Select one or more from each category)

Same categories as lunch
In addition, two fruits of your choice and one glass of lowfat milk.

Some scientists have proposed that the imbalance between the amounts of free radicals produced and available amounts of vitamins A, C and E and selenium may be responsible for normal aging processes (e.g., more free radicals and fewer vitamins and selenium may increase the rate of aging). If this is the case, the presence of sufficient amounts of these nutrients may reduce the damage and thereby reduce the rate of some degenerative changes associated with aging, especially in the brain.

COMMON WAYS IN WHICH VITAMINS AND OTHER NUTRIENTS ARE MISUSED

1. In recent years many nutrition books have been published, and some contain erroneous information regarding doses and dose-schedules for supplementary nutrients. Thus, careful selection of a book by which to prepare your diet guidelines is important. Make sure that the credentials of the authors include research, patient care, and teaching expertise in the area of vitamins and nutrition.

2. Base your estimate of vitamins and nutrients for daily consumption on your needs and check with a physician who is knowledgeable in this area to see if your estimates are reasonable.

3. Do not buy any vitamins or nutrients which are not fully described on the label.

4. Do not take excessive amounts of nutrients that will make you sick. Some nutrition books have suggested that one should increase the doses in the beginning until some kind of sickness is manifested, then decrease the doses until a comfortable level is reached. This is very dangerous, as some nutrients in large amounts can cause irreversible damage.

5. If you have further questions, consult experts who are actively involved in research, teaching, or patient care (see pages 76–87).

The above considerations will make your efforts to improve your health and to reduce the risk of cancer more effective and less expensive.

CHAPTER

3.

Treating Cancer

WHAT IS THE CURRENT STATUS OF CANCER THERAPY?

Before discussing the role of vitamins in the treatment of cancer, it is important to understand the nature of cancer cells and the current status, usefulness and limitations of different kinds of therapy.

Are all cells of a cancer similar? If all cells of a cancer were similar, treating cancer would be easy, because one therapeutic agent would be sufficient to kill all of the cells. Unfortunately, cancer cells are very complex in the sense that there are many different kinds of cells within the same cancer. Therefore, a variety of drugs which have different modes of action are commonly used in treating cancer. This approach kills more cancer cells than would be killed by a single agent.

It has been repeatedly observed that cancer cells may become very unresponsive to *all* therapeutic agents after a period of good initial response. This is because almost all of the agents used to treat cancer also *cause* cancer themselves. During treatment these agents produce many biochemical changes among those cancer cells which are not killed and make them "super cancer cells." Such "super cancer cells" cannot be killed, even by a more poisonous chemical.

Thus, tumors contains cells many of which are different from each other. Some differences are inherent (i.e., they are present before treatment), whereas other differences are

57

acquired (i.e., they are produced by treatment agents). From those observations it seems clear that the complexity of tumor cells increases during the treatment phase and that no single agent may ever be sufficient to cure tumors.

BENEFITS AND LIMITATIONS OF VARIOUS TREATMENTS

Current cancer therapies include surgery, chemotherapy, radiation therapy, heat therapy and treatment with monoclonal antibodies (a kind of protein which is supposed to kill specific cancer cells without killing normal cells). Frequently surgery is used in combination with chemotherapy and radiation, or in combination with chemotherapy, radiation and heat. Monoclonal antibodies are being used as an experimental drug in the treatment of certain cancers. The usefulness and limitations of each of these agents are discussed below.

Surgery

Surgery is one of the most commonly used procedures in the treatment of solid cancers that are accessible to such treatment. However, many cancer sites are not accessible and even when they are, minute, invisible tumors are likely to be left in the body. Nevertheless, surgery is considered one of the best available approaches to cancer therapy because it does not significantly increase the risk of developing new cancer or noncancer diseases later.

Chemotherapy

Many toxic chemicals are used extensively in treating cancer, frequently in combination with surgery and radiation. Almost all of them kill both cancer cells and normal cells, cause severe illness, destroy the body's immune defense system, and increase the risk of new cancer among patients who survive more than five years.

It has been reported that the incidence of leukemia (blood cancer) and solid tumors among the survivors of chemotherapy and radiation therapy is about 10 percent. However, the observation periods upon which this figure is based are usually no more than 10 years after completion of treatment. According to present knowledge, the risk of additional leukemia may not increase any further, but the risk of developing new solid cancers and noncancerous diseases persists up to 30 years or more after treatment. In spite of these limitations, chemotherapy must be used until better treatment methods are established.

Radiation Therapy

Radiation is commonly used in treating human cancer. It is frequently used in combination with surgery or chemotherapy, or both. Like chemotherapy, radiation produces toxic effects. It kills both normal and cancer cells, causes severe illness, destroys the body's immune defense system, and increases the risk of new cancer among those who survive. Generally the time interval between radiation exposure and detection of new tumors is about 10 years for leukemia and up to 30 years or more for solid tumors. The risk of developing noncancerous diseases also persists long after completion of treatment (usually more than 15 years). In spite of these limitations, radiation must be used until better treatment methods are established.

Heat Therapy

Generally temperatures of 42°–43°C (107.6°–109.4°F) are used in heat therapy, primarily for the purpose of controlling local tumors. However, raising whole body temperature from

37 °C (98.6 °F) to 42 °C or 43 °C would be lethal. Heat is frequently used in combination with radiation therapy. This approach has provided occasional relief for some patients when other treatment methods were ineffective, but in general results have been disappointing. Some recent laboratory experiments suggest that the use of high temperatures (42 °–43 °C) in combination with radiation may actually increase the incidence of radiation-induced cancer. Because of these limitations, the use of high temperatures (over 41 °C, or 105.8 °F) cannot be considered in designing long-term treatment strategies for human cancer. However, the use of heat therapy at a lower temperature (40 °C, or 104 °F), in combination with nontoxic chemicals, may be of some value in treating human cancer, because the whole-body temperature can be raised from 37 ° to 40 °C without toxic effects.

Monoclonal Antibody Therapy

Cancer cells are used in the preparation of monoclonal antibodies, a kind of immune protein. It is assumed that such monoclonal antibodies will kill all cancer cells which have receptors for these antibodies. Unfortunately not all cancer cells have receptors for these antibodies, and so some are not killed. Thus, the usefulness of antibodies in treating cancer is limited. Nevertheless, if even a small percentage of cancer cells are killed by such a selective means, continued research and development of this method is justified.

Current treatment methods have produced increasing numbers of long-term survivors of early stage diseases, such as Hodgkin's disease, childhood leukemia, Wilms' tumor (kidney), cervical cancer, prostate cancer, neuroblastoma, retinoblastoma (eye tumor), and melanoma. The risk of future consequence exists in these "cured" patients. In most other cancers, current treatment agents have been less effective.

Delayed Consequences of Cancer Therapies

Based on a five-year survival rate, significant progress has been made in the treatment of some cancers. But if one considers recent indications of an increased risk of developing new cancer and noncancer diseases, one becomes concerned about the consequences and adequacy of current methods of treatment. Noncancerous diseases that may afflict survivors include the following:

Aplastic anemia—if the bone marrow was involved during therapy.

Paralysis—if the spinal cord was involved during therapy.

Cataract—if one or both eyes were involved during therapy.

Reproductive failures—if the gonads were involved during therapy.

Necrosis—in nondividing organs such as the brain, liver and muscle cells, if they were involved during therapy.

Retardation of growth—if the patient was a child.

It should be pointed out that both radiation and chemotherapy can produce further disease many years after treatment. Because of these potential risks, newer approaches to cancer treatments which utilize nontoxic agents *must* be developed. However, it should be emphasized that current methods of treatment *must be continued*, despite potential risks, until better therapies are developed.

BETTER METHODS OF CANCER TREATMENT

The best ways to treat cancer would be to transform all cancer cells to normal cells, or to kill all cancers cells without killing normal cells, or both. In order to achieve the first goal, we need to understand the basic steps involved in maintaining the regular features of normal cells and the basic events by which normal cells *become* cancer cells. In order to achieve the second goal, we need to identify nontoxic substances that kill cancer cells without killing normal cells. If one considers the evolution of cancer cells in the body, nontoxic agents that change cancer cells to normal cells and that kill only tumor cells may, in theory, be found. For example, the transformation from normal cells to cancer cells probably occurs more frequently than we realize; however, these newly formed cancer cells do not always develop into detectable cancer, possibly because the body has an elaborate defense system, which includes the immune system. When cancer cells escape the body's defense system, they continue to grow and become detectable. If we can identify those substances that constitute the body's defense system, it will be possible to kill tumor cells selectively without killing normal cells.

WHY VITAMINS?

Numerous laboratory experiments indicate that there are several nontoxic and naturally occurring substances that change some cancer cells back to normal cells and that kill cancer cells *without* killing normal cells. These include vitamins A, C and E. The following sections describe the importance of vitamins, alone and in combination with currently used tumor therapeutic agents, in treating cancer.

Laboratory studies have led to clinical trials of vitamins, primarily A, C and E, in treating certain advanced human cancers. Preliminary results show that high doses of each of these vitamins reduce the growth of tumors. At this time it is not known whether a combination of vitamins A, C and E is more effective in reducing tumor growth than the vitamins individually. Laboratory experiments suggest that vitamins may markedly improve cancer treatment in the following ways:

1. Reducing tumor growth without affecting normal cells.
2. Transforming some cancer cells to normal cells.
3. Enhancing the cell-killing effects of currently used chemotherapeutic agents, radiation and heat.
4. Reducing some of the toxic side effects certain chemotherapeutic agents have on normal cells.
5. Stimulating the body's immune defense system.

The extent and type of effect of vitamins depend upon the type, form, dosage and method of administration, as well as the type and stage of tumor. The importance of individual vitamins in treating cancer is discussed below.

Vitamin A

The recurrence of melanoma (a kind of skin cancer) after surgical removal of the primary tumor is high (30–75 percent), depending upon the stage of the cancer. It has been reported that the combination of BCG vaccine with vitamin A (100,000 I.U. per day) for 18 months slightly increases the period of disease-free time in melanoma (stages 1 and 2) more than BCG vaccine alone. The side effects of this treatment included dry skin and mild depression.

A pronounced beneficial effect of 13-cis-retinoic acid, an analog of vitamin A, on cutaneous T-cell lymphoma (mycosis fungoides) was observed. Eight of twelve patients responded well, with four showing a nearly complete cure of the disease. Beneficial effects of vitamin A were also observed on patients with epithelial tumors. Some epithelial tumor cells are resistant to vitamin A; the reasons for their resistance are unknown. Vitamin A was ineffective in treating nonepithelial cancer. Further studies are needed to evaluate the role of vitamin A alone in the treatment of human cancers. It is certain that vitamin A by itself will not be sufficient in the treatment of advanced cancer.

Vitamin C

Although vitamin C has been shown to reduce the growth of animal tumors, its role in treating human cancer has become controversial. Cameron and Pauling have reported that the administration of high doses of sodium ascorbate (5–10 grams per day) increases the survival of patients with advanced cancer. These patients were either treated minimally or not treated at all with conventional therapies. Other scientists have reported that high doses of vitamin C were ineffective in improving the survival of patients with terminal cancer. These patients were treated extensively with radiation and chemotherapy before being given vitamin C. Thus, the difference in results may be due to the fact that in the patients of Cameron and Pauling the tumor contained cells which were sensitive to vitamin C; whereas in the other patients the tumors contained cells which became more complex because of treatment with chemicals and radiation, and thus were resistant to vitamin C. Therefore, the treatment of cancer with vitamin C alone may possibly be of some value when it is given before radiation of chemotherapy.

A recent study in Japan has reported that local infusion of sodium ascorbate with copper and glycyl-glycyl-histidine, a peptide, caused complete regression of osteosarcoma (bone cancer) in a patient. This observation is very exciting and calls for further research. It should be pointed out, however, that vitamin C alone may never be sufficient in the treatment of advanced cancer.

Vitamin E

Laboratory experiments have shown that vitamin E causes some cancer cells to revert to normal and that it inhibits the growth of several other cancer cells. However, cancer cells that are resistant to vitamin E do exist, and the reasons for their resistance are unknown. The extent and type of effect depend upon the form of cancer and the form of vitamin E; vitamin E succinate is more potent than other forms. In a recent clinical trial, high doses of vitamin E (alpha-tocopherol) were used to treat human neuroblastoma that had become unresponsive to all standard therapeutic agents. It has been reported that more than 50 percent of these patients showed partial regression of their cancer.

It should be pointed out that the vitamin E (alpha-tocopherol) that is being used may not be the most potent form of vitamin E. In view of the fact that those who received vitamin E therapy were all patients who were terminally ill in spite of receiving all available therapy, the preliminary results noted above should be considered encouraging. Further preclinical and clinical studies using vitamin E succinate must be performed.

Some other clinical studies suggest that administering high doses of vitamin E is also useful in patients with chronic cystic mastitis, the most common benign tumor of the female breast.

Because of the presence of different kinds of cells in a cancer and because vitamins A, C and E have, in part, different ways of acting, the combination of these three vitamins may be more effective in the treatment of cancer than the individual vitamins. However, no animal or human studies have been performed to test this concept.

Vitamin B$_6$

Several animal studies have reported that the supplemental vitamin B$_6$, one of the vitamins of vitamin B complex, enhances the growth of cancer and that the restriction of vitamin B$_6$ retards it. The relevance of this observation for human cancer is not known at this time. Nevertheless, supplemental vitamin B$_6$ should be avoided during treatment of cancer.

Vitamin D

Some recent laboratory experiments have shown that 1-alpha-hydroxyvitamin D_3 reduces the growth of certain cancers (melanoma, a kind of skin cancer; hepatoma, a liver cancer; myeloid leukemia, a kind of blood cancer). Further studies are needed to evaluate the role of vitamin D in the treatment of cancer.

Modification of the effects of tumor therapeutic agents by vitamins A, C and E: Results of animal experiments indicate that vitamins A, C and E modify (increase or decrease) the effects of therapeutic agents (chemicals, radiation and heat) on cancer cells. The extent of modification depends upon the types of tumor cells, the types of vitamins, and the types of therapeutic agents.

Cancer therapeutic agents can be grouped into the following categories: radiation, surgery, chemotherapeutic agents, naturally occurring anticancer agents, and heat. The enhancement of the effects of radiation, chemotherapeutic agents and heat on tumor cells by vitamins is discussed below.

Vitamin A enhances the beneficial effects of radiation and chemotherapy: Animal studies suggest that vitamin A and beta-carotene inhibit the growth of breast cancer in animals. The combination of vitamin A and radiation was more effective than the individual agents. Cancers were completely cured in mice given both vitamin A and radiation. Beta-carotene was equally effective. The combination of cyclophosphamide, a commonly used cancer-therapeutic chemical, with vitamin A or beta-carotene produced a greater regression of tumor growth than did the cyclophosphamide treatment alone. Combining vitamin A with certain tumor-therapeutic agents may improve the management of cancer, but it has not been tested in human beings. It is important to remember that cancer cells which are resistant to the combined effects of vitamin A and a tumor-therapeutic agent exist in the same tumor.

Vitamins C enhances the beneficial effects of radiation: It has been shown that vitamin C increases the effects of radiation on animal neuroblastoma cells, but not on animal glioma cancer cells. Vitamin C in combination with radiation enhances the survival of mice with ascitis (cells in fluid of the abdominal cavity) more than that produced by radiation treatment alone. It has been reported that vitamin C protects Chinese hamster ovary cells against radiation damage. Further studies are needed on these topics.

Vitamin E enhances the beneficial effects of chemotherapeutic agents and radiation: Most currently used chemotherapeutic agents destroy the body's defense system and make people terribly sick. These agents are not normally present in the body but are manufactured synthetically. They kill normal cells as well as cancer cells. It has been reported that vitamin E, in combination with currently used chemotherapeutic agents, is more effective on tumor cells than the individual agents. However, it must be pointed out that the extent of this kind of effect of vitamin E depends upon the type of cancer and the type of chemotherapeutic agent. If this result is found in human beings, the addition of vitamin E to currently used treatments using chemotherapeutic agents may markedly improve their effectiveness in treating human cancer. It is also possible that the doses of chemotherapeutic agents required for effective treatment may be markedly reduced, and the risk of severe sickness decreased. Extensive studies are in progress to evaluate the role of vitamin E in enhancing the effectiveness of currently used chemotherapies.

Laboratory experiments have shown that vitamin E acetate and vitamin E succinate increase the effects of radiation on neuroblastoma and glioma (brain tumor). Vitamin E has been shown to protect normal tissue against radiation damage. Furthermore, recent studies show that high doses of vitamin E succinate enhance the effects of radiation on tumor cells, whereas low doses of vitamin E are ineffective in enhancing the effects of radiation.

These observations suggest that whenever vitamin E is combined with radiation, high doses of vitamin E should be used; otherwise, the use of vitamin E may be ineffective. It must be pointed out that the above observations have **not** been tested extensively on either animal or human cancer. Also, laboratory experiments have shown that there are cancer cells that are resistant to the combined effects of vitamin E and radiation.

If vitamins C and E enhance the effects of radiation on human cancer, the addition of these vitamins to radiation therapy may markedly improve its effectiveness and may even reduce the long-term risk of developing new cancer and noncancer diseases. Extensive studies are in progress to test these possibilities.

Vitamin E enhances the beneficial effects of naturally occurring anticancer agents. The use of toxic drugs in treating human tumors continues to be emphasized, but it cannot be accepted as the ideal kind of therapy.

An alternative approach must be developed. Recent studies suggest that it may be possible to treat human cancer by using high doses of nontoxic, naturally occurring substances. These agents at higher concentrations turn some cancer cells into normal cells or reduce the growth of tumors without affecting the normal cells, or both. Some of these are vitamins A, C and E (all discussed previously).

In addition to vitamins, two naturally occurring substances, adenosine $3'$, $5'$ cyclic monophosphate (cAMP) and butyric acid, have been shown to produce an anticancer effect in the laboratory. cAMP is a chemical substance which is found in all cells of the body. Several laboratory experiments have suggested that a defect in the cAMP system may be associated with the formation of cancer cells. If this is the case, then the correction of this defect should convert cancer cells to normal cells. Indeed, when this problem in the cAMP system is corrected by using another chemical, the cancer cells of some tumors such as neuroblastoma (a childhood cancer that occurs primarily in the abdomen), melanoma (a kind of skin cancer), oat cell carcinoma (a kind of lung cancer), glioma (a kind of brain cancer), and pheochromocytoma (a kind of adrenal cancer) become normal cells. As expected, not all cells are converted to normal cells by correcting the above defect. Therefore, an additional study must be performed to find out how the remaining cancer cells can be changed to normal cells. The fact that cancer cells can be converted to normal cells by utilizing cAMP-stimulating agents is very exciting, but the usefulness of this concept in treating human cancer has been tested in only one type of cancer (neuroblastoma). The addition of cAMP-stimulating agents to the treatment protocols for advanced neuroblastoma has shown some encouraging results.

Butyric acid, a small size fatty acid, occurs in the human body. In cancer experiments, butyric acid is used as sodium butyrate (non-acidic form). Numerous laboratory experiments have shown that sodium butyrate at high doses also converts some cancer cells (erythroid leukemia, a cancer of blood cells) to normal cells. In addition, it kills some other cancer cells without killing normal cells (for example, neuroblastoma, sarcoma, glioma and melanoma cells). As expected, not all cancer cells are killed by sodium butyrate. We have to find out the ways by which some of the remaining cancer cells can be killed or be converted to normal cells. Limited human studies suggest that sodium butyrate at high doses (up to 10 grams a day) is nontoxic and produces beneficial effects in some patients with advanced neuroblastomas and erythroid leukemia. However, many more experiments are needed before its usefulness for human cancer can be assessed.

Studies show that vitamin E enhances the antitumor effects of cAMP and sodium butyrate on neuroblastoma, glioma and melanoma cells under laboratory experimental conditions. The extent of vitamin E-induced enhancement depends upon the form of cancer and the type of agent. Thus, it is very encouraging to note that we now have at least five naturally occurring substances, namely vitamins A, C and E, cAMP and butyric acid, that have been shown to produce anticancer effects on experimental systems and on certain types of advanced human cancer when used as a single agent. The combined effects of these agents on laboratory experimental systems have not been evaluated.

Vitamin E enhances the beneficial effects of heat. During the last 10 years extensive experiments and clinical studies of the effects of heat alone, or in combination with X rays and certain chemicals, have been conducted. However, the results of clinical trials have been disappointing because the temperatures required to kill cancer cells are 42°–43°C and are fatal when the whole body is raised to these temperatures. Even in the treatment of local lesions, heat has been of very limited value; in addition, high temperatures (42°–43°) increase the potential of X rays to cause cancer. The use of heat in the treatment of tumors will continue to be restricted to local lesions until the cell-killing effects of heat can be achieved at temperatures near 40°C, which are not toxic to the whole body. Vitamin E succinate in combination with heat at 40°C was more effective than the individual agents in reducing the growth of neuroblastoma cells. (Vitamin C did not enhance the effect of heat on the neuroblastoma, glioma and melanoma cells studies.)

Vitamin C can enhance or reduce the effects of chemotherapeutic agents and naturally occurring anticancer agents. Nontoxic concentrations of sodium ascorbate increase the growth inhibitory effect of several chemotherapeutic agents and some naturally occurring substances such as cAMP and sodium butyrate. Unlike vitamin E, sodium ascorbate reduces the killing effects of chemotherapeutic agents such as DTIC and methotrexate. These results suggest that whenever a combination of vitamin C and a chemotherapeutic agent is considered, it must be based on experimental results that support the desired effect. The addition of vitamin C without such a rationale may be ineffective or even counterproductive.

Vitamin C's ability to modify the effects of currently used tumor-therapeutic agents has not been tested adequately on either animal or human cancer. One study has shown, however, that sodium ascorbate combined with CCNU (a commonly used chemotherapeutic agent) enhances the survival of mice with leukemia twofold, in comparison with results obtained when CCNU is used alone. Further animal studies are needed before these findings can be applied to human cancer.

Vitamins E and C can reduce the side effects of currently used chemotherapeutic agents. Several animal studies have shown that vitamin E may reduce adriamycin-induced cardiac toxicity and skin ulcers. Vitamin E has also been shown to protect against bleomycin-induced lung fibrosis. Additional studies have established that vitamin E succinate is more effective than vitamin E acetate in treating cancer. It has been reported that vitamin E protects the immune system against the destructive effect of some chemotherapeutic agents, such as Adriamycin, mitomycin C, and 5-fluorouracil. It has also been reported that sodium ascorbate significantly reduced Adriamycin-induced heart damage in mice and guinea pigs. The relevance of these results to human beings is being tested in Japan.

At this time these findings cannot be readily extrapolated to human cancer. Human studies are needed for confirmation.

From available laboratory results, it appears that adding

vitamins A, C and E to currently used treatments may greatly improve their effectiveness. However, it must be emphasized that the use of vitamins in combination with tumor-therapeutic agents must be done with a biological rationale; otherwise, the addition of vitamins may not be effective and may even be harmful. The role of other vitamins in combination with currently used tumor-therapeutic agents remains to be evaluated.

DESIGNING A NUTRITION AND LIFESTYLE PROGRAM FOR THOSE WHO ARE IN REMISSION AFTER BEING TREATED FOR CANCER

What is remission? During remission cancer cannot be detected by known technologies, either because there are very few cancer cells left or because there are no cancer cells at all.

How is remission achieved? Surgery, extensive chemotherapy and radiation therapy can produce a remission in certain types of tumors, if they are detected at early stages. These include neuroblastoma, a childhood tumor; Wilms' tumor, a childhood kidney tumor; Hodgkin's disease, a tumor of blood cells; certain childhood leukemias; breast cancer; cervical cancer; prostate cancer; and melanoma.

What are the consequences of classical cancer therapies? There are four possible major consequences:

1. The person becomes free of cancer.
2. The original cancer may recur, generally within 5 to 10 years, because a few cancer cells were left after treatment and they could not be eliminated by the body's defense system.
3. The person may be cured of the original cancer, but may develop new tumors 10–30 years after treatment.

4. The person may develop noncancerous diseases such as paralysis, reproductive failure, increased aging, reduction in growth, aplastic anemia, cataract, and necrosis of several vital organs (brain, liver muscle, etc.)

Some laboratory experiments suggest that it is possible to influence consequences 2, 3, and 4 above by designing an appropriate diet, together with appropriate amounts of supplemental vitamins A, C and E, selenium, and restricted amounts of vitamin B_6. However, there are no human data yet to support these possibilities.

INTERIM DIET GUIDELINES

1. Eat more fresh fruits and vegetables, especially those rich in vitamins A, C and E for breakfast, lunch and dinner (see Table 9 for selection guidelines).
2. Eat one or two carrots a day.
3. Eat only whole wheat bread and cereals. Do not overbake any wheat preparations to the point that they become dark.
4. Eat minimally refined rice preparations.
5. Take moderate amounts of fish (unless you are a vegetarian) after removing the skin and fatty parts. Fish is a rich source of selenium.

INTERIM SUPPLEMENTARY NUTRITION GUIDELINES

At this time there are no human data that permit the estimation of doses of vitamins and minerals which would be most effective in preventing or delaying the recurrence of cancer after remission has been achieved. Based on laboratory research, the following vitamin doses and dose schedules are suggested.

Vitamin A

15,000 I.U. per day, divided into two doses, taken orally, once in the morning and once in the evening, each dose containing 5,000 I.U. retinol or retinyl acetate, and 2,500 I.U. of beta-carotene.

Vitamin C

Up to 2 grams per day, taken orally, divided into four doses, in the form of sodium ascorbate or calcium ascorbate.

Vitamin E

300 I.U. per day, divided into two doses, taken orally, once in the morning and once in the evening, each dose containing 100 I.U. of vitamin E acetate or vitamin E succinate, and 50 I.U. of vitamin E (alpha-tocopherol).

Vitamin B$_6$

Do not take supplemental vitamin B$_6$. Limit the intake of vitamin B$_6$ through diet.

Selenium

100 micrograms per day, divided into two doses, taken orally, once in the morning and once in the evening. Selenium must be taken in the form of organic selenium, such as yeast selenium. Inorganic selenium, such as sodium selenite, is absorbed very poorly from the small intestine.

INTERIM LIFESTYLE GUIDELINES

1. Reduce your fat consumption by 30 percent of your current level.
2. Eat less cholesterol. Egg yolk is very rich in cholesterol, so whenever eggs are eaten, remove about 50 percent of the yolk.
3. Reduce all meat consumption markedly.
4. Eat less charcoal-broiled, smoked, preserved and cured meat. Whenever they are consumed, make sure to take 250 milligrams of vitamin C and 100 I.U. of vitamin E (alpha-tocopherol).
5. Eat pickled products (fruits, vegetables, fish and meat) as little as possible.
6. Reduce your consumption of alcohol markedly.
7. AVOID TOBACCO COMPLETELY and, until you quit, never mix smoking with drinking alcohol.
8. Reduce your consumption of regular or decaffeinated coffee and tea (not more than one or two cups a day).
9. Reduce your consumption of cold drinks that contain caffeine or saccharine, or both.
10. Avoid consuming excessive amounts of cheese.
11. Drink only lowfat milk. Lowfat yogurt and lowfat cottage cheese are also recommended.

What results may be expected from such a program?

1. Prevention of cancer recurrence.
2. Marked delay of cancer recurrence.
3. Prevention or delay of onset of new cancer.

It is to be emphasized that the above suggestions regarding diet, supplemental vitamins, selenium and lifestyle are based only on animal studies, some indirect human studies, and the known safe limits of the nutrients are discussed.

Major Studies on Vitamins, Nutrition, and Cancer

STUDIES ON CANCER TREATMENT

1. Dr. F.L. Meyskens Jr. (treatment of human cancer, vitamin A), University of California Cancer Center, Orange, CA 92668, USA.

2. Dr. G.E. Goodman (treatment of human cancer, vitamin A), Tumor Institute of Swedish Hospital, Seattle, Washington 98104, USA.

3. Dr. G. Mathe (treatment of human cancer, vitamin A), Service des Maladies Sanguines et Tumorales, Institut de Cancerologie et d'Immunogenetique (INSERM U-50), Hôpital, Paul-Brousse, F-94804, France.

4. Dr. G.J.S. Rustin (treatment of human cancer, vitamin A), Department of Medical Oncology, Charing Cross Hospital, London, W68 RF, England.

5. Dr. W.J. Uphouse (treatment of human cancer, vitamin A), Cancer Center of Hawaii, 1236 Lauhala Street, Rm 301, Honolulu, Hawaii 96813, USA.

6. Dr. L. Itri (treatment of human cancer, vitamin A), Hoffmann—La Roche, Inc., Nutley, New Jersey 07110, USA.

7. Dr. N.J. Lowe (treatment of human cancer, vitamin A), Division of Dermatology, School of Medicine, University of California at Los Angeles, Los Angeles, California 90024, USA.

8. Dr. M.M. Black (treatment of human cancer, vitamins A and E), Department of Pathology, New York Medical College, Valhalla, New York 10595, USA.

9. Dr. W.L. Robinson (treatment of human cancer, vitamin A), Division of Oncology, Department of Medicine, University of Colorado Health Sciences Center, Denver, Colorado 80262, USA.

10. Dr. G.L. Peck (treatment of human cancer, vitamin A), Dermatology Branch, National Cancer Institute, Building 10, Bethesda, Maryland 20205, USA.

11. Dr. W. Bollag and Dr. H.R. Hartmann (treatment of human cancer, vitamin A), Pharmaceutical Research Development, F. Hoffmann-La Roche & Co., Ltd., CH-4002, Basel, Switzerland.

12. Dr. L. Pauling (treatment of human cancer, vitamin C), 440 Page Mitt Road, Palo Alto, California 94306, USA.

13. Dr. F. Morishige (treatment of human cancer, vitamin C), Tachiarai Hospital, 842-1, Yamaguma Miwa-machi, Asakura-gun, Fukuoka, 838, Japan.

14. Dr. A. Hanck (treatment of human cancer, vitamin C), Unit of Social and Preventive Medicine, University of Basel, Switzerland.

STUDIES ON HUMAN CANCER PREVENTION

15. Dr. T. Moon (vitamin A), Cancer Center, University of Arizona Health Sciences Center, Tucson, Arizona 85724, USA.

16.   Dr. J. Li (vitamins A, C and E), Department of Epidemiology and Cancer Institute, Chinese Academy of Medical Sciences, Beijing, People's Republic of China.

17.   Dr. L.M. DeLuca, Dr. W. DeWys, Dr. P. Greenwald (vitamins A, C and E), National Cancer Institute, Bethesda, Maryland 20205, USA.

18.   Dr. C. Hennekens (vitamin A), Harvard Medical School, Boston, Massachusetts 02115, USA.

19.   Dr. R.L. Phillips (diets), Loma Linda Studies School of Health, Loma Linda University, Loma Linda, California 92350, USA.

20.   Dr. C. Mettlin (vitamin A), Roswell Park Memorial Institute, 666 Elm Street, Buffalo, New York 14263, USA.

21.   Dr. S. Graham (vitamin A), Departments of Sociology and Social and Preventive Medicine, State University of New York at Buffalo, Buffalo, New York 14214, USA.

22.   Dr. G. Kvale (vitamins A, C and E), Institute of Hygeine and Social Medicine, University of Bergen, Norway.

23.   Dr. M. Micksche (vitamin A), Institute of Cancer Research, University of Vienna, Ludwig Boltzmann Institute for Clinical Oncology, Municipal Hospital, Lainz-Vienna, Austria.

24.   Dr. R. Doll (vitamins A, C and E), Imperial Cancer Research Fund, Cancer Epidemiology Unit, 9 Keble Road, Oxford, OX13QG, England.

25.   Dr. R. Peto (vitamins A, C and E), Imperial Cancer Re-

search Fund Cancer Unit, Nuffield, Department of Clinical Medicine, Radcliffe Infirmary, Oxford, OX26HE, England.

26. Dr. E.L. Wynder (diets), American Health Foundation, Valhalla, New York 10595, USA.

27. Dr. J. Wylie-Rosett (vitamin A), Department of Community Health, Albert Einstein College of Medicine, 1300 Morris Park Avenue, Bronx, New York 10461, USA.

28. Dr. A.J. Tuyns (vitamin C), Unit of Analytical Epidemiology, International Agency for Research on Cancer, 15—Cours Albert Thomas, F69372, Lyon, Cedex 08, France.

29. Dr. R. Burton (vitamins A, C and E), Research Institute for Social Security, Helsinki, Finland.

30. Dr. P. Helms (vitamins A, C and E), Institute of Hygiene, Aarhus, Denmark.

31. Dr. L. Bjerrum and Dr. A. Paerregaard (vitamins A, C and E), St. Elizabeth Hospital, Copenhagen, Denmark.

32. Dr. J.H. Cummings and Dr. W.J. Branch (vitamins A, C and E), Dunn Clinical Nutrition Center, Addenbrook's Hospital, Trumpington Street, Cambridge, England.

33. Dr. S.A. Broitman (alcohol and nutrition), Departments of Pathology and Microbiology, Boston University School of Medicine, Boston, Massachusetts 02118, USA.

34. Dr. B.S. Reddy and Dr. J.H. Wisburger (fibers), Naylor Dana Institute for Disease Prevention, American Health Foundation, Valhalla, New York 10595, USA.

35.   Dr. T. Campbell (diets and nutrition), Division of Nutritional Sciences, Cornell University, Ithaca, New York 14850, USA.

LABORATORY STUDIES

36.   Dr. E. Seifter (vitamin A), Department of Surgery, Albert Einstein College of Medicine, 1300 Morris Park Avenue, Bronx, New York 10461, USA.

37.   Dr. R.C. Moon (vitamin A), Laboratory of Pathophysiology, Life Sciences Building, IIT Research Institute, Chicago, Illinois 60616, USA.

38.   Dr. T.K. Basu (vitamins A and C), Department of Food and Nutrition, University of Alberta, Edmonton, Alberta, T6G2M8, Canada.

39.   Dr. L. Santamaria (vitamin A), C. Golgi Institute of General Pathology, University of Pavia, Piazza Botta n. 10. I-27100 Pavia, Italy.

40.   Dr. R.W. Shearer (vitamin A), 2017 East Beaver Lake Drive, Issaquah, Washington 98027, USA.

41.   Dr. N.T. Telang (vitamins), Laboratory of Molecular Biology and Virology, Memorial Sloan-Kettering Cancer Center, New York, New York 10021, USA.

42.   Dr. S. Takase (vitamins), Departments of Nutrition and Biochemistry, Shizuoka Women's University, 409 Yada, Shizuoka-City, Shizuoka 422, Japan.

43.   Dr. T.J. Slaga (vitamins A, C and E), The University of Texas System of Cancer Center, Science-Park Research Division, Smithville, Texas 78957, USA.

44. Dr. D. Flavin (vitamins A, C and E), The Nutrition Foundation, 9319 Old George Town Road, Bethesda, Maryland 20814, USA.

45. Dr. P. Newberne (vitamin E and selenium), Massachusetts Institute of Technology, 50 Ames Street, Cambridge, Massachusetts 02139, USA.

46. Dr. K.N. Prasad (vitamins E and C), Center for Vitamin and Cancer Research, Department of Radiology, University of Colorado Health Sciences Center, Denver, Colorado 80262, USA.

47. Dr. E. Bright-See (vitamins E and C) and Dr. H. Newmark (vitamins), Ludwig Institute for Cancer Research, 9 Earl Street, Toronto, Ontario, M4Y1M4, Canada.

48. Dr. I. Sadek (vitamins A and E), Zoology Department, Alexandria University, Cairo, Egypt.

49. Dr. R.P. Tengerdy (vitamin E), Department of Microbiology, Colorado State University, Fort Collins, Colorado 80523, USA.

50. Dr. S.V. Kandarkar (vitamin A), Cancer Research Institute, Parel Bombay, India.

51. Dr. D.G. Hendricks (vitamins), Departments of Nutrition and Food Sciences, Utah State University, Logan, Utah 84322, USA.

52. Dr. R. Lotan (vitamin A), M.D. Anderson Hospital and Tumor Institute, Department of Tumor Biology, Houston, Texas 77030, USA.

53. Dr. Y.M. Yang (vitamin E), M.D. Anderson Hospital and Tumor Institute, University of Texas System Cancer Center, Houston Texas 77030, USA.

54. Dr. L.W. Wattenberg (vitamin E and other antioxidants), Department of Pathology, University of Minnesota, Minneapolis, Minnesota 55455, USA.

55. Dr. B.P. Sani (vitamin C), Kettering Meyer Laboratory, Southern Research Institute, Birmingham, Alabama 35203, USA.

56. Dr. A.M. Jetten (vitamin A), National Institute of Environmental Health Sciences, Research Triangle, North Carolina 27709, USA.

57. Dr. E.P. Norkus (vitamin C), Dr. H. Bhagavan (vitamins A, C and E) and Dr. L. Machlin (vitamin E), Hoffmann-La Roche, Inc., Nutley, New Jersey 07110, USA.

58. Dr. R. Gol-Winkler (vitamin C), Laboratorie de Chimie Medicale, Institut de Pathlogie, Universite de Liege, Batiment B-23, B-4000, Start Tilman Par Liege 1, Belgium.

59. Dr. C.H. Park (vitamin C), Department of Medicine, University of Kansas Medical Center, Kansas City, Kansas 66103, USA.

60. Dr. V.P. Sethi (vitamin C), Oncology Research Center, Bowman Gray School of Medicine of Wake Forest University, Winston-Salem, North Carolina 27103, USA.

61. Dr. J.A. Eisman (vitamins), University of Melbourne, Respiratory General Hospital, Heidelberg, Victoria, 3084, Australia.

62. Dr. M. Hozumi (vitamins A and E), Department of Chemotherapy, Saitama Cancer Center, Research Unit, Saitama—362, Japan.

63. Dr. L.H. Chen (vitamins C and E), Departments of Nutrition and Food Sciences, University of Kentucky, Lexington, Kentucky 40506, USA.

64. Dr. H. Fortmeyer (vitamins), Tieversuchsanlage des Klinikum der J.W. Goeth-universitat, Theodor Stern Ka 1 7, D-6000, Frankfurt, West Germany.

65. Dr. M.B. Sporn (vitamin A), Laboratory of Chemoprevention, National Cancer Institute, Bethesda, MD 20892, USA.

66. Dr. F. Chytil (vitamin A), Departments of Biochemistry and Medicine, Vanderbilt University, School of Medicine, Nashville, Tennessee 37240, USA.

67. Dr. A.T. Diplock (vitamin E and selenium), Department of Biochemistry, Royal Free Hospital, School of Medicine, University of London, London, England.

68. Dr. A. Trichopoulou (vitamins), Departments of Nutrition and Biochemistry, Athens School of Hygiene, Leof Alexandria 196, GR-11521, Athens, Greece.

69. Dr. G.N. Schrauzer (selenium), Department of Chemistry, University of California at San Diego, La Jolla, California 92093, USA.

70. Dr. J.W. Thanassi (vitamin B_{12}), Department of Biochemistry, University of Vermont, College of Medicine, Burlington, Vermont 05405, USA.

71. Dr. G.P. Tryfiates (vitamin B_{12}), Department of Biochemistry, West Virginia University, School of Medicine, Morgantown, West Virginia 26506, USA.

72. Dr. D.G. Zaridze (vitamins), WHO, Centre Internationale de Recherche sur le Cancer, 150 cours Albert-Thomas 69732, Lyon, Cedex 08, France.

73. Dr. M.H. Zile (vitamins), Departments of Food Sciences and Human Nutrition, Michigan State University, East Lansing, Michigan 48824, USA.

74. Dr. H. Fujuki (vitamins) and Dr. T. Sugimura (vitamins), National Cancer Center Research Institute, 1-1, Tsukijil, 5- Chome, Chou-ku, Tokyo, 104, Japan.

75. Dr. A.E. Rogers (vitamins), Departments of Nutrition and Food Sciences, Massachusetts Institute of Technology, Cambridge, Massachusetts 02139, USA.

76. Dr. T.R. Breitmann (vitamins), National Center Institute, Bethesda, Maryland 20205, USA.

77. Dr. P.B. McCay (vitamin E, antioxidants), Oklahoma Medical Foundation, Oklahoma City, Oklahoma 73104, USA.

78. Dr. J.C. Bertram (vitamins), Grace Cancer Drug Center, Roswell Park Memorial Institute, 666 Elm Street, Buffalo, New York 14263, USA.

79. Dr. F.E. Jones (vitamin A), Department of Surgery, College of Medicine, 8700 West Wisconsin Avenue, Milwaukee, Wisconsin 53226, USA.

80. Dr. B.S. Alam (vitamin A), Department of Biochemistry,

Louisiana State University Medical Center, New Orleans, Louisiana 70119, USA.

81. Dr. G. Shklar (vitamin E), Departments of Oral Medicine and Oral Pathology, Harvard School of Dental Medicine, Boston, Massachusetts 02115, USA.

82. Dr. D.M. Klurfeld (vitamin A), The Wistar Institute of Anatomy and Biology, 36th Street at Spruce, Philadelphia, Pennsylvania 19104, USA.

83. Dr. S.J. Van Rensburg (vitamin A), National Research Institute for Nutritional Diseases, Tygerberg, 7505, South Africa.

84. Dr. D.M. Disorbo (vitamin B_6), Oncology Research Laboratory, Nassau Hospital, Mineola, New York 11501, USA.

85. Dr. Y. Tomita (vitamin A), Department of Public Health, Kurume University School of Medicine, Kurume-830, Japan.

86. Dr. A.R. Kennedy (protease inhibitors and antioxidants), Department of Radiation Oncology, University of Pennsylvania Medical School, 3400 Spruce Street, Philadelphia, Pennsylvania, 19104, USA.

87. Dr. K.K. Carroll (fat), Department of Biochemistry, University of Western Ontario, London, Ontario, N6A5C1, Canada.

88. Dr. B.N. Ames (diets and vitamins), Department of Biochemistry, University of California, Berkeley, California 94720, USA.

89. Dr. I. Emerit (antioxidants), Université de Pierre et Marie Curie, Paris, France.

90. Dr. D. Schmahl (vitamin C), Institute of Toxicology and Chemotherapy, German Cancer Research Center, Heidelberg, West Germany.

91. Dr. Y.S. Hong (vitamins A, C and E), Ewha Women's University, College of Medicine, Seoul, South Korea.

92. Dr. C. Ip (vitamin E and selenium), Department of Breast Surgery, Roswell Park Memorial Institute, Buffalo, New York 14263, USA.

93. Dr. L.G. Israels (vitamin K), Manitoba Institute of Cell Biology, University of Manitoba, Winnipeg, Manitoba, Canada.

94. Dr. R.G. Ham (nutrients), Department of Molecular Cellular and Developmental Biology, University of Colorado, Boulder, Colorado 80309, USA.

95. Dr. J.P. Berry (selenium), SC 27 Inserm, Laboratoire de Biophysique, Faculté de Medecine, 94010, Creteil, France.

96. Dr. M. Sakaguchi (fat), Department of Surgery, Kansai Medical University, 1 Fumizono, Moriguchi, Osaka, 570, Japan.

97. Dr. S.M. Przybyszewski (vitamin E and other antioxidants), Department of Biochemistry, Institute of Hematology, 00-957, Warsaw, Poland.

98. Dr. C. Beckman (vitamin E), Biology Department, Concordia University, Montreal, Quebec, Canada.

99.   Dr. M. Menkes and Dr. G. Comstock (vitamin E), The Johns Hopkins Training Center for Public Health Research, Hagerstown, Maryland 21740, USA.

100.   Dr. J.T. Salomen (selenium and human cancer), Research Institute of Public Health, Department of Community Health, University of Kuopio, 70211 Kuopio-1, Finland.

101.   Dr. M.G. Le (alcohol and human cancer), Institute Gustave Roussy, Villejuif, France.

102.   Dr. K.A. Poirier and Dr. J.A. Milner (selenium and animal cancer), Department of Food Science, Division of Nutritional Sciences, University of Illinois, Urbana, Illinois 61801, USA.

Further Reading

Diet, Nutrition and Cancer, National Academy of Sciences Press, Washington, D.C., 1982.

Meyskens, F.L. Jr., and Prasad, K.N. (Editors). *Modulation and Mediation of Cancer by Vitamins,* pp. 1–348, Basel, Karger Press, 1983.

Prasad, K.N. (Editor). *Vitamins, Nutrition and Cancer,* pp. 1–400, Basel, Karger Press, 1984.

Cameron, E., and Pauling, L. *Vitamin C and Cancer.* New York, Warner Books, 1981.

Higginson, J., and Muir, C.S. Environmental carcinogenesis: Misconceptions and limitations to cancer control. *Journal of National Cancer Institute.* 63: 1291–1298, 1979.

Wynder, E.L., and Gori, G.B. Contribution of the environment to cancer incidence: An epidemiologic exercise. *Journal of National Cancer Institute.* 58: 825–832, 1977.

Bjelke, E. Dietary vitamin A and human lung cancer. *International Journal of Cancer.* 15: 562–565, 1975.

Prasad, K.N., and Edwards-Prasad, J. Effect of tocopherol (vitamin E) acid succinate on morphological alteration and growth inhibition in melanoma cells in culture. *Cancer Research.* 43: 550–555, 1982.

Benedict, W.F., Wheatley, W.L., and Jones, P.A. Inhibition of chemically induced morphological transformation and reversion of the transformed phenotype by ascorbic acid in C3H/10T½ cells. *Cancer Research* 40: 2796–2801, 1980.

Lotan, R. Effect of vitamin A and its analogs (retinoids) on normal and neoplastic cells. *Biophysica Acta.* 605: 33–91, 1981.

Sporn, M.B. Retinoids and carcinogenesis. *Nutritional Reviews.* 35: 65–69, 1977.

Kurek, M.P., and Corwin, L.M. Vitamin E protection against tumor formation by transplanted murine sarcoma cells. *Nutrition and Cancer.* 4: 128–139, 1982.

Griffin, A.C. Role of selenium in the chemoprevention of cancer. *Advances in Cancer Research.* 29: 419–442, 1979.

Graham, S., Mettlin, C., Marshall, J., Priore, R., Rzepka, T., and Shedd, D. Dietary factors in the epidemiology of cancer of the larnyx. *American Journal of Epidemiology.* 113: 675–680, 1981.

Jain, M., Cook, G.M., Davis, F.G., Grace, M.G., Howe, G.R., and Miller, A.B. A case control study of diet and colorectal cancer. *International Journal of Cancer.* 26: 757–768, 1980.

Reddy, B.S. Dietary macronutrients and colon cancer. In: *Vitamins, Nutrition and Cancer.* Editor: Prasad, K.N. pp. 212–230, Basel, Karger Press, 1984.

Broitman, S.A. Relationship of ethanolic beverages and ethanol to cancers of the digestive tract. In: *Vitamins, Nutrition and Cancer.* Editor: Prasad, K.N. pp. 195–211, Basel, Karger Press, 1984.

Schrauzer, G.N. Selenium in nutritional cancer prophylaxis: An update. In: *Vitamins, Nutrition and Cancer.* Editor: Prasad, K.N. pp. 240–250, Basel, Karger Press, 1984.

Flavin, D.F., and Kolbye, A.C. Jr. Nutritional factors with a potential to inhibit critical pathways of tumor promotion. In: *Modulation and Mediation of Cancer by Vitamins.* Editors: Meyskens F.L., Jr., and Prasad, K.N. pp. 24–38, Basel, Karger Press, 1983.

Boutwell, R.K. Biology and biochemistry of the two-step model of carcinogenesis. In: *Modulation and Mediation of Cancer by Vitamins.* Editors: Meyskens, F.L., Jr., and Prasad, K.N. pp. 2–9. Basel, Karger Press, 1983.

Slaga, T.J. Multistage skin carcinogenesis and specificity of inhibitors. In: *Modulation and Mediation of Cancer by Vitamins.* Editors: Meyskens, F.L., Jr., and Prasad, K.N. pp. 10–23, Basel, Karger Press, 1983.

Cook, M.G., and McNamara, P. Effect of dietary vitamin E on dimethylhydrazine-induced colonic tumor in mice. *Cancer Research.* 40: 1329–1331, 1980.

Doll, R., and Peto R. The cause of cancer. Quantitative estimates of available risks of cancer in the United States today. *Journal of National Cancer Institute.* 66: 1192–1308, 1981.

Sporn, M.B., Roberts, A.B., and Goodman, D.S., (Editors). *The Retinoids.* Academic Press, Orlando, 1984.

Shamberger, R.J., Baughman, F.F., Kalchert, S.L., et al. Carcinogen-induced chromosomal breakage decreased by antioxidants. *Proceedings of National Academy of Sciences.* 70: 1461–1463, 1973.

Wylie-Rosett, J., Romney, S., Slagle, S., Wassertheil-Smoller, S.,

Miller, G.L., Palan, P.R., Lucido, D.J., and Duttagupta, C. Influence of vitamin A on cervical dysplasia and carcinoma in-situ. *Nutrition and Cancer.* 6:49–57, 1984.

Zedek, M.S., and Lipkin, M. (Editors). *Inhibition of tumor induction and development.* New York, Plenum Press, 1981.

Palgi, A. Vitamin A and lung cancer. *Nutrition and Cancer.* 6: 105–119, 1984.

Odukoya, O., Hawach, F., and Shaklar, G. Retardation of experimental oral cancer by topical vitamin E. *Nutrition and Cancer.* 6: 98–104, 1984.

Disorbo, D.M., and Nathanson, L. High dose pyridoxal supplemented culture medium inhibits the growth of a human malignant melanoma cell line. *Nutrition and Cancer.* 5:10–15, 1983.

Klurfeld, D.M., Aglow, E., Tepper, S.A., and Kritcheusky, D. Modification of dimethylhydrazine-induced carcinogenesis in rats by dietary cholesterol. *Nutrition and Cancer.* 5:16–23, 1983.

Kummet, T., Moon, T.E., and Meyskens, F.L. Jr., Vitamin A. Evidence for its preventive role in human cancer. *Nutrition and Cancer.* 5: 96–106, 1983.

Jones, F.E., Komorowski, R.A., and Condon, R.E. The effects of ascorbic acid and butylated hydroxyanisole in the chemoprevention of 1, 2-dimethylhydrazine-induced large bowel neoplasm. *Journal of Surgical Oncology.* 25: 54–60, 1984.

Ames, B.N. Dietary carcinogens and anticarcinogens. *Science.* 221: 1256–1264, 1983.

Newbern, P.M., and Suphakarn, V. Nutrition and cancer. A review with emphasis on the role of vitamin C and vitamin E and selenium. *Nutrition and Cancer.* 5: 107–117, 1983.

Black, M.M., Zachrau, R.E., Dion, A.S., and Katz, M. Stimulation of prognostically favorable cell-mediated immunity of breast cancer patients by high dose vitamin A and vitamin E. In: *Vitamins, Nutrition and Cancer.* Editor: Prasad, K.N. pp. 134–146, Basel, Karger Press, 1984.

Prasad, K.N., and Rama, B.N. Modification of the effect of pharmacological agents on tumor cells in culture by vitamin C and vitamin E. In: *Modulation and Mediation of Cancer by Vitamins.* Editors: Meyskens, F.L. Jr., and Prasad, K.N., pp. 244–257, Basel, Karger Press, 1983.

Kennedy, A.R. Prevention of radiation transformation in-vitro. In: *Vitamins, Nutrition and Cancer.* Editor: Prasad, K.N., pp. 166–179, Karger Press, Basel, 1984.

Meyskens F.L., Jr., Prevention and treatment of cancer with vitamin A and retinoids. In: *Vitamins, Nutrition and Cancer.* Editor: Prasad, K.N., pp. 266–273, Basel, Karger Press, 1984.

Recommended Dietary Allowances, 9th Edition, Washington, D.C., National Academy of Sciences, 1980.

Prasad, K.N. Differentiation of neuroblastoma cells in culture. *Biological Reviews.* 50: 129–165, 1975.

Rosenberg, R.N. Neuroblastoma and glioma cell cultures in studies of neurologic functions: The clinician's Rosetta Stone. *Neurology.* 27: 105–108, 1977.

Haffke, S.C., and Seeds, N.W. Neuroblastoma: The *E. coli* of neurobiology. *Life Sciences.* 16: 1649–1658, 1975.

Prasad, K.N. Therapeutic potentials of differentiating agents in neuroblastomas. In: *Biology of Cancer (2).* Editors: Mirand, E.A., Hutchinson, W.B., and Mihich, E., pp. 75–89, New York, Alan R. Liss, 1983.

Imashuku, S., Todo, S., Amano, T., Mizukawa, K., Sugimoto, T., and Kusonoki, T. Cyclic AMP in neuroblastoma, ganglioneuroma, and sympathetic ganglia. *Experientia.* 33: 1507, 1977.

Imashuku, S., Sugano, T., Fukiwara, K., Todo, S., Shinjiro, T., Ogita, S., and Goto, Y. Intra-aortic prostaglandin E1 (PGE1) infusion, papaverine and multiagent chemotherapy in disseminated neuroblastoma. *Cancer Research.* 23: 478a, 1983.

Prasad, K.N. Butyric acid: a small fatty acid with diverse biological functions. *Life Sciences.* 27: 1351–1358, 1980.

Novogrodsky, A., Dvir, A., Sholnik, T., Stenzel, K.H., Rubin, A.L., and Zaizov, R. Effect of polar organic compounds on leukemic cells: Butyrate induced partial remission of acute myelogenous leukemia in a child. *Cancer.* 51: 9–11, 1983.

Wald, N.J., Boreham, J., Hayward, J.L., and Bulbrook, R.D. Plasma retinol, beta-carotene and vitamin E levels in relation to the future risk of breast cancer. Prospective studies involving 5,000 women. *British Journal of Cancer.* 49: 321–324, 1984.

Kinlen, L.J., and Mcpherson, K. Pancrease cancer and coffee and tea consumption. A case-control study. *British Journal of Cancer.* 49: 93–96, 1984.

Ohkoshi, M., Ohta, H., and Ito, M. Effect of vitamin B_2 on tumorigenesis of 3-methylcholanthrene in the mouse. *Gann* (Japan). 73: 105–107, 1982.

Lambooy, J.P. Influence of riboflavin antagonists on azodye hepatoma induction in the rat. *Proceedings of the Society for Experimental Biology and Medicine.* 153: 532–535, 1976.

Le, M.G., Hill, C., Kramar, A., and Flamant, R. Alcoholic beverage consumption and breast cancer in a French case-control study. *American Journal of Epidemiology.* 120: 350–357, 1984.

Salonen, J.T., Alfthan, G., Huttunen, J.K., and Puska, P. Association between serum selenium and the risk of cancer. *American Journal of Epidemiology.* 120: 342–349, 1984.

Menkes, M. and Constock, G. Vitamin A and E and lung cancer. *American Journal of Epidemiology.* 120: 491 (abstract), 1984.

Yasunaga, et al. Protective effect of vitamin E against immunosuppression induced by Adriamycin, mitomycin C, and 5-fuorouracil in mice. *Nippon Geka Hokan* (Japan). 52: 591–601, 1983.

Sram, R.J., Samkova, I., and Hola, N. High dose ascorbic acid prophylaxis in workers occupationally exposed to halogenated ethers. *Journal of Hygiene, Epidemiology, Microbiology, and Immunology.* 27: 305–318, 1983.

Tryfiates, G.P. Control of tumor growth by pyridoxine restriction or treatment with an antivitamin agent. *Cancer Detection and Prevention.* 4: 159–164, 1981.

Mihich, E.; Rosen, F.; and Nichol, C.A. The effect of pyridoxine deficiency on a spectrum of mouse and rat tumors. *Cancer Research.* 19: 1244–1248, 1959.

Tryfiates, G.P. and Prasad, K.N. (Editors). *Nutrition, Growth and Cancer,* New York, Alan R. Liss, 1988.

INDEX